Navigation in Oral and Maxillofacial Surgery

Seyed Alireza Parhiz • Jeffrey N. James
Shohreh Ghasemi
Mohammad Hosein Amirzade-Iranaq
Editors

Navigation in Oral and Maxillofacial Surgery

Applications, Advances, and Limitations

Springer

Editors
Seyed Alireza Parhiz
Department of Oral
& Maxillofacial Surgery
Tehran University of Medical Sciences
Tehran, Iran

Shohreh Ghasemi
Oral and Maxillofacial Surgery
Augusta University
Marrieta, GA, USA

Jeffrey N. James
Oral and Maxillofacial Surgery
Augusta University
Augusta, GA, USA

Mohammad Hosein Amirzade-Iranaq
Universal Network of Interdisciplinary
Research in Oral and Maxillofacial
Surgery (UNIROMS)
Universal Scientific Education and Research
Network (USERN)
Tehran, Iran

ISBN 978-3-031-06222-3 ISBN 978-3-031-06223-0 (eBook)
https://doi.org/10.1007/978-3-031-06223-0

This Springer imprint is published by the registered company Springer Nature Switzerland AG
The registered company address is: Gewerbestrasse 11, 6330 Cham, Switzerland

Foreword

Over the past three decades, we have witnessed major technological advances in the management of patients requiring oral or maxillofacial reconstructive surgery. This is primarily a result of (1) the development of computed tomography (CT) imaging for improved diagnosis and treatment planning; (2) rigid internal fixation, for more predictable outcomes and rapid return to function; (3) dental implant support prosthetic rehabilitation,; (4) microvascular free tissue transfer, resulting in immediate return to form and function compared to pedicled flaps; (5) computer-aided design/computer-aided manufacturing, which facilitated custom implants, guide stents and cutting guides for better accuracy; and (6) intraoperative navigation and mobile CT imaging, which provide added precision, especially for complex problems with difficult surgical access. With these improvements come higher endpoints to achieve both aesthetic and functional reconstructive outcomes and a heretofore unrealized standard of care.

In particular, the use of three-dimensional data obtained from CT images for virtual surgical planning (VSP), stereolithographic and rapid model prototyping, and intraoperative navigation has provided an important solution for the problem of reestablishing facial symmetry and accurately repositioning skeletal or composite tissue constructs into ideal antero-posterior, vertical, and sagittal relationships. These relationships should ideally result in favorable facial proportions and orthognathic jaw relationships that facilitate successful implant-supported prosthetic rehabilitation. The use of virtual surgical planning and biomodels obtained from CT data as well as intraoperative navigation based on these virtual plans has undoubtedly aided the assessment of patients in three dimensions leading to improved outcomes. It has also helped to reduce intraoperative surgical time with all its associated benefits such as shorter graft ischemia time and lower operating room costs. With VSP and intraoperative navigation, immediate implant placement planning is also feasible with the ultimate outcome being the introduction of the "Jaw in a day" concept, in which jaw reconstruction, implant and immediate prosthesis placement are all performed during the same operation following the ablative surgery. All of these new advances are rapidly being incorporated into new standards of care that require multidisciplinary teams to most effectively manage patients with congenital or developmental craniofacial deformity, craniomaxillofacial trauma, head and neck pathology, and dentoalveolar bone and tooth loss.

Against this backdrop, Dr. Alireza Parhiz, Dr. Mohmmad Hossein Amirzade-Iranaq, Dr. Jeffrey N. James, and Dr. Shohreh Ghasemi and their colleagues led by Drs. Ahmadiyan, Politis, Reddy, Kim, G Mauer, and Tohme provide a comprehensive textbook for managing the most common reconstructive challenges in the oral and maxillofacial region, with an emphasis on intraoperative navigation. This textbook will serve as an important point of reference for continued improvements in treatment paradigms that will lead to even better outcomes for patients with congenital, developmental, or acquired deformity, and we all look forward to these future advancements.

R. Bryan Bell
Division of Surgical Oncology
Radiation Oncology and Cancer Programs
Head and Neck Cancer Program
Providence Cancer Institute-Oregon
Portland, OR, USA

Surgical Oncology Research
Earle A. Chiles Research Institute
a Division of Providence Cancer Institute
Portland, OR, USA

Preface

Science makes tools; tools will assist practitioners; finally, assisted procedures result in more satisfaction and improved outcomes. Surgical navigation technology is one of the advances demonstrating various applications in various surgical specialties. The head and neck region is a critical area that requires a vast amount of precision and caution, which is where the navigation technology reveals to be of assistance.

In 2010 when visiting ZOL hospital in Belgium for a study opportunity, I became familiar with navigation technology. Our experiences with this technology for orthognathic and foreign object removal surgeries under the supervision of Prof. Politis in the Department of Oral and Maxillofacial Surgery were promising and inspiring.

Years later, after returning to Iran, I had the opportunity to meet the professional team managed by Prof. Ahmadian, the first designer and manufacturer of navigation systems in Iran. After consultations, I started to work on developing navigation technology for oral and maxillofacial surgeries in the Sina Hospital, Tehran, Iran. Continuous advances in various aspects of this technology, especially in registration, encouraged our team, including surgeons and engineers, to successfully perform over a hundred navigation-assisted oral and maxillofacial surgeries in recent years.

The amount of valuable experiences and knowledge gathered these years by our team encouraged us to organize, evaluate, and document the evidence as a useful source for other oral and maxillofacial surgeons to enjoy using navigation systems in their practice.

The current edited volume aims to cover navigation advances in various surgical specialties including, but not limited to, trauma surgery, implant surgery, and orthogenetic surgery. Chapters will also discuss surgical pathology as well as guided surgeries.

Our invited authors are all well-known scientists and surgeons with valuable experience in using navigation technology for oral and maxillofacial surgeries.

With these words, I would like to especially thank Prof. Politis for accepting our invitation to enrich this book with his valuable knowledge and experience. Also.

Prof. Ahmadian for critical evaluation of navigation technology for clinical use from an engineer's point of view.

My sincere gratitude is dedicated to my coeditors for their efforts, Dr. Jeffrey N. James, Dr. Ghasemi, and Dr. Amirzade-Iranaq.

Navigation in Oral and Maxillofacial Surgery tries to be comprehensive, precise, and a "must-have" resource for clinicians in the fields of oral and maxillofacial surgery, otorhinolaryngology-head and neck surgery, trauma surgery, and plastic surgery, as well as researchers and postgraduate students in related fields.

Tehran, Iran — Seyed Alireza Parhiz
Augusta, GA, USA — Jeffrey N. James
Marietta, GA, USA — Shohreh Ghasemi
Tehran, Iran — Mohammad Hosein Amirzade-Iranaq

Contents

Contributors

Alireza Ahmadian Department of Medical Physics and Biomedical Engineering, Faculty of Medicine, Tehran University of Medical Sciences (TUMS), Tehran, Iran

Research Centre of Biomedical Technology and Robotics (RCBTR), Advanced Medical Technologies and Equipment Institute (AMTEI), Tehran University of Medical Sciences, Tehran, Iran

Amirhossein Ahmadian Department of Mechanical and Aerospace Engineering, University of California, Los Angeles, CA, USA

Maryam Jalili Aziz Department of Medical Physics and Biomedical Engineering, Faculty of Medicine, Tehran University of Medical Sciences (TUMS), Tehran, Iran

Research Centre of Biomedical Technology and Robotics (RCBTR), Advanced Medical Technologies and Equipment Institute (AMTEI), Tehran University of Medical Sciences, Tehran, Iran

Ritesh Bhattacharjee Department of Oral & Maxillofacial Surgery, College of Dentistry, Texas A&M University, Dallas, TX, USA

Oral & Maxillofacial Surgery, Baylor University Medical Center, Dallas, TX, USA

Mahmood Dashti Med Spa, Esfahan, Iran

Parastoo Farnia Department of Medical Physics and Biomedical Engineering, Faculty of Medicine, Tehran University of Medical Sciences (TUMS), Tehran, Iran

Research Centre of Biomedical Technology and Robotics (RCBTR), Advanced Medical Technologies and Equipment Institute (AMTEI), Tehran University of Medical Sciences, Tehran, Iran

Beomjune Kim Department of Head and Neck/Microvascular Reconstructive Surgery, Cancer Treatment Centers of America in Atlanta, Part of City of Hope, Newnan, GA, USA

Saeedeh Navaei Lavasani Research Centre of Biomedical Technology and Robotics (RCBTR), Advanced Medical Technologies and Equipment Institute (AMTEI), Tehran University of Medical Sciences, Tehran, Iran

Ghida Lawand Prosthodontics and Esthetic Dentistry Department, Faculty of Dentistry, Saint Joseph University, Beirut, Lebanon

Tian Lei Department of oral and maxillofacial surgery, College of Stomatology, The Fourth Military Medical University, Xi'an, Shaanxi, China

Reihaneh G. Mauer Periodontist at Mauer Periodontics & Implant Dentistry, LLC, Fort Myers, FL, USA

Ebrahim Najafzadeh Department of Medical Physics and Biomedical Engineering, Faculty of Medicine, Tehran University of Medical Sciences (TUMS), Tehran, Iran

Research Centre of Biomedical Technology and Robotics (RCBTR), Advanced Medical Technologies and Equipment Institute (AMTEI), Tehran University of Medical Sciences, Tehran, Iran

Constantinus Politis Oral and Maxillofacial Surgery—Imaging and Pathology Research Group, Department of Imaging and Pathology, University of Leuven, Leuven, Belgium

Department of Oral & Maxillofacial Surgery, University Hospitals Leuven, Leuven, Belgium

Likith Reddy Department of Oral & Maxillofacial Surgery, College of Dentistry, Texas A&M University, Dallas, TX, USA

Oral & Maxillofacial Surgery, Baylor University Medical Center, Dallas, TX, USA

Medical Education, College of Medicine, Texas A& M University, Dallas, TX, USA

Cesar Rivera Department of Oral & Maxillofacial Surgery, College of Dentistry, Texas A&M University, Dallas, TX, USA

Oral & Maxillofacial Surgery, Baylor University Medical Center, Dallas, TX, USA

Aida Shadrav UCLA School of Dentistry, Los Angeles, CA, USA

Eman Shaheen Oral and Maxillofacial Surgery—Imaging and Pathology Research Group, Department of Imaging and Pathology, University of Leuven, Leuven, Belgium

Department of Oral & Maxillofacial Surgery, University Hospitals Leuven, Leuven, Belgium

Yi Sun Oral and Maxillofacial Surgery—Imaging and Pathology Research Group, Department of Imaging and Pathology, University of Leuven, Leuven, Belgium

Department of Oral & Maxillofacial Surgery, University Hospitals Leuven, Leuven, Belgium

Hani Tohme Digital Dentistry Unit, Clinical Director of Postgraduate Program - Removable Prosthodontics Department, Faculty of Dentistry, Saint Joseph University, Beirut, Lebanon

Andrew Yampolsky Department of Oral and Maxillofacial Surgery, Sidney Kimmel Medical College, Thomas Jefferson University Hospital, Philadelphia, PA, USA

Waleed Zaid Department of Oral and Maxillofacial Surgery, Louisiana State University Health Sciences Center—School of Dentistry, New Orleans, LA, USA

Fundamentals of Navigation Surgery

Alireza Ahmadian, Parastoo Farnia, Ebrahim Najafzadeh, Saeedeh Navaei Lavasani, Maryam Jalili Aziz, and Amirhossein Ahmadian

1 History of Navigation System

Nowadays, the medical and healthcare industries are very different from those in previous years, thanks to emerging advances in technology. In the medical field, technology is increasingly playing a critical role in almost all procedures, from diagnosis to treatment. One of the main areas of technological advances is related to medical imaging technologies, which have made substantial contributions to medicine over the past several decades. However, when it comes to surgical treatment, translation of the preoperative images to the operation field is a challenging procedure for surgeons. The Image-Guided Surgery (IGS) system is one of the most widely acknowledged technologies in the area of surgery, from simple biopsy to complex surgeries [1].

IGS systems operate in a manner similar to global positioning satellites (GPS) used by automobiles and mobile phones. Just as it is impossible to envision routing without a car or a mobile GPS today, it will certainly be impossible to imagine surgery without the use of IGS systems in the coming years. In IGS, surgical tools are

A. Ahmadian (✉) · P. Farnia · E. Najafzadeh · M. J. Aziz
Department of Medical Physics and Biomedical Engineering, Faculty of Medicine, Tehran University of Medical Sciences (TUMS), Tehran, Iran

Research Centre of Biomedical Technology and Robotics (RCBTR), Advanced Medical Technologies and Equipment Institute (AMTEI), Tehran University of Medical Sciences, Tehran, Iran
e-mail: Ahmadian@tums.ac.ir

S. N. Lavasani
Research Centre of Biomedical Technology and Robotics (RCBTR), Advanced Medical Technologies and Equipment Institute (AMTEI), Tehran University of Medical Sciences, Tehran, Iran

A. Ahmadian
Department of Mechanical and Aerospace Engineering, University of California, Los Angeles, CA, USA

S. A. Parhiz et al. (eds.), *Navigation in Oral and Maxillofacial Surgery*,
https://doi.org/10.1007/978-3-031-06223-0_1

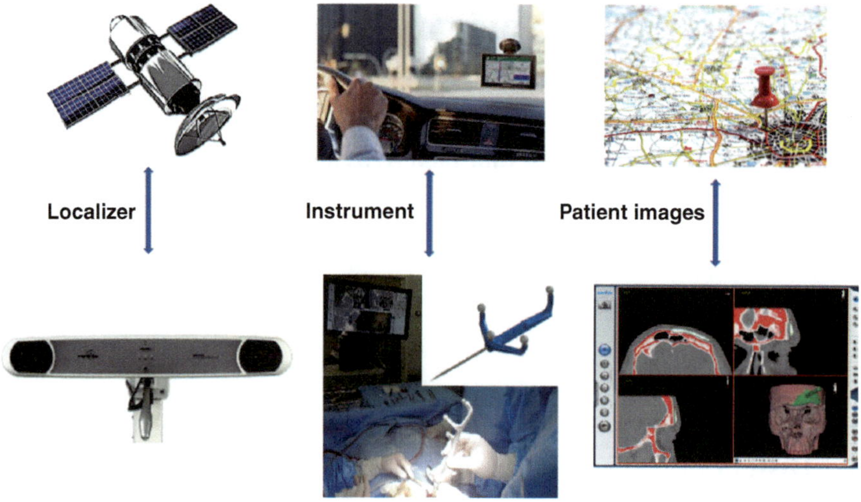

Fig. 1 Corresponding components of GPS and IGS. The surgical IGS is similar to the GPS systems commonly used in mobile phones and has three main components: a localizer, which functions similarly to a satellite in space; a surgical instrument or pointer like the GPS unit in the vehicle which emits track waves; and preoperative data which is analogous to a roadmap

tracked in real-time procedure and displayed in the correct location and orientation on preoperative images to directly guide the procedure, as shown in Fig. 1.

This technology enables the surgeon to precisely localize pathological tissue and relevant anatomical structures during a less invasive and safer real-time procedure. As a result, it has become a recognized standard of surgery in a variety of surgical specialties, including neurosurgery, spine, orthopedic, ears, nose, and throat (ENT), and craniomaxillofacial (CMF). Real-time feedback for surgeons, improving patient safety and outcomes, minimally invasive surgery, preservation of tissue function, decreasing operating and recovery time, reducing subjective workload, improving surgeon maneuvers during surgery to assist them in identifying anatomical structures, and improving visualization of the operative field are all advantages of IGS systems [2–9].

As obvious, images play a critical role in the evolution of navigation systems. Without images, image-guided surgery and navigation would be useless. As so, the history of navigation is inextricably linked to the history of medical imaging. Medical imaging began on November 8, 1895, with the accidental discovery of X-ray at the University of Würzburg, Germany, by physicist Wilhelm Conrad Röntgen. Two weeks after discovering X-ray, Röntgen captured the first image of his wife's hand, Anna Ludwig (Fig. 2).

The findings of Röntgen were published on December 28, 1895. Only 8 days after his publication, the first image-guided intervention was performed by J. H. Clayton from England. Clayton used the X-ray to determine the location of the industrial sewing needle and then performed needle removal surgery on the

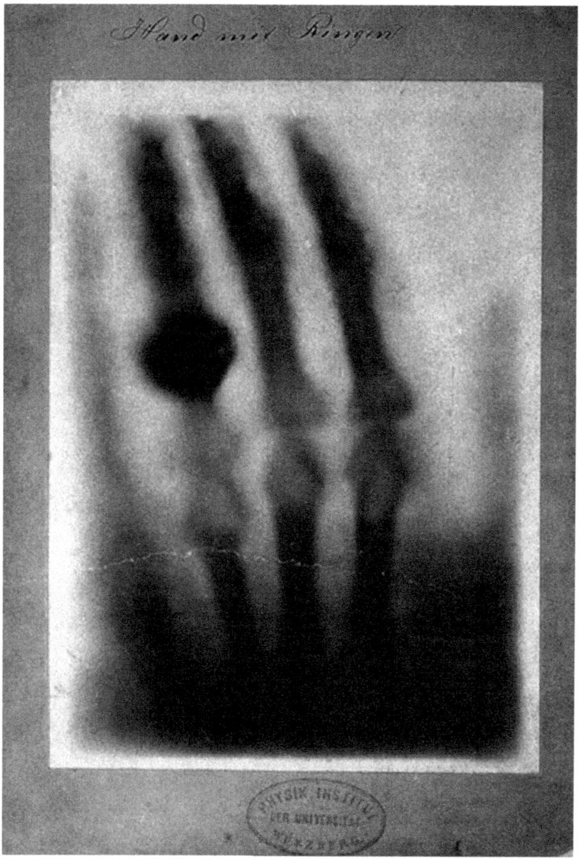

Fig. 2 The first known X-ray image taken by Röntgen of his wife's hand, Anna Ludwig, captured on December 22, 1895 [10]

worker's hand. Then, X-ray imaging by producing a two-dimensional (2D) projection of three-dimensional (3D) anatomy onto film was used in the removal of foreign objects/bullets during surgery [1].

In 1972, an incredible invention of Sir Godfrey Hounsfield of EMI Laboratories and Allan Cormack of Tufts University, computerized axial tomography (CAT), later known as computed tomography (CT), was publicly announced (Fig. 3). This imaging modality acquires projections from many directions to create tomographic images of the body in cross-sections (slice-by-slice), and therefore, each tissue appears separately from other tissues in the image [11].

This revolutionary in imaging helped neurosurgeons to use CT imaging to track the entry of a needle into the patient's brain to ensure precise lesion targeting, in combination with a three-dimensional stereotaxic frame as a mechanical guide in the shape of a huge metal box mechanically attached to the patient's skull to stabilize the head during a procedure (Fig. 4). In other words, this system was used to more precisely pinpoint specific body parts by utilizing attached landmarks on the patient's head.

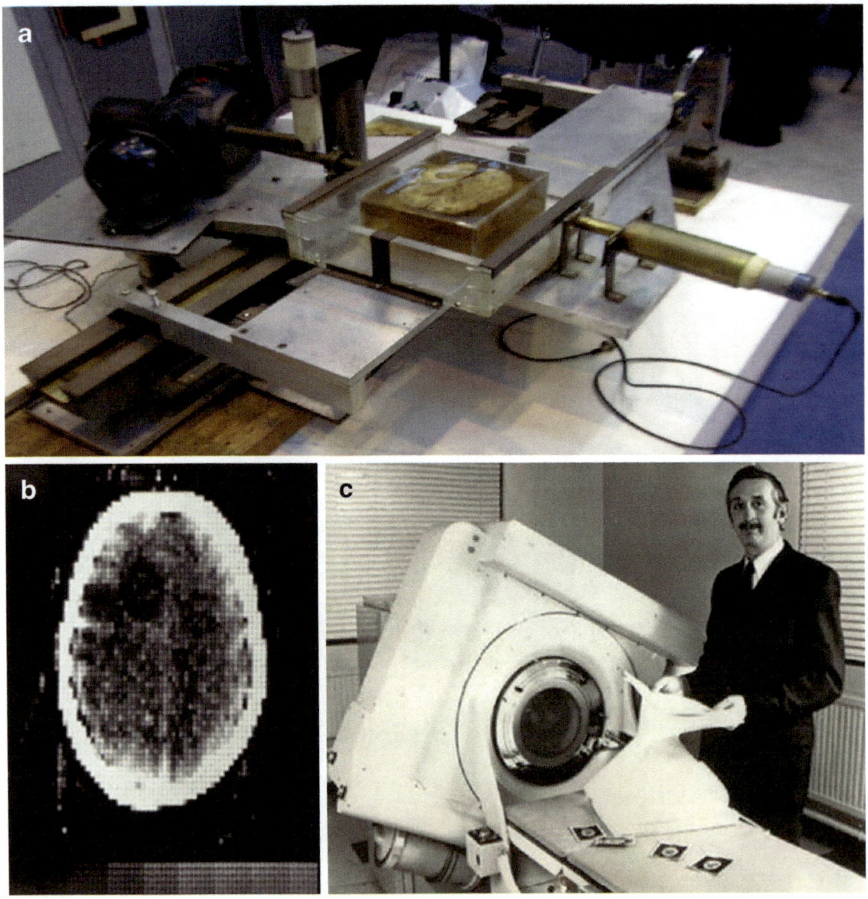

Fig. 3 (**a**) The first CAT scanner prototype (http://www.impactscan.org/CThistory.htm). (**b**) The first clinical scan captured with EMI CAT prototype on October 1, 1971 (image size was 80 × 80 matrix) (http://www.impactscan.org/CThistory.htm). (**c**) Hounsfield with the first commercial head CT scanner (https://catalinaimaging.com/history-ct-scan/)

On the other hand, Horsley and Clarke described the first stereotactic frame in 1908 for making lesions in the central nervous system of animals. Following them, Aubrey Mussen designed a stereotactic apparatus for use on humans (Fig. 5a); as a result, the first human stereotaxic frame was built in 1918 in London [13]. However, no procedures were carried out with this instrument until Robert Hayne and Frederic Gibbs used a stereotaxic frame for depth electroencephalography in 1947. The structure of frames has been improved since their first construction, becoming more precise and lighter. The Stereotaxic frame improved reproducibility of patient setup, accuracy, and speed of operation procedures (Fig. 5b). However, using a stereotaxic frame is an invasive procedure as the frame should be screwed onto the patient's skull, which is not comfortable for the patient [14]. Therefore, the researchers were looking for an alternative frameless solution.

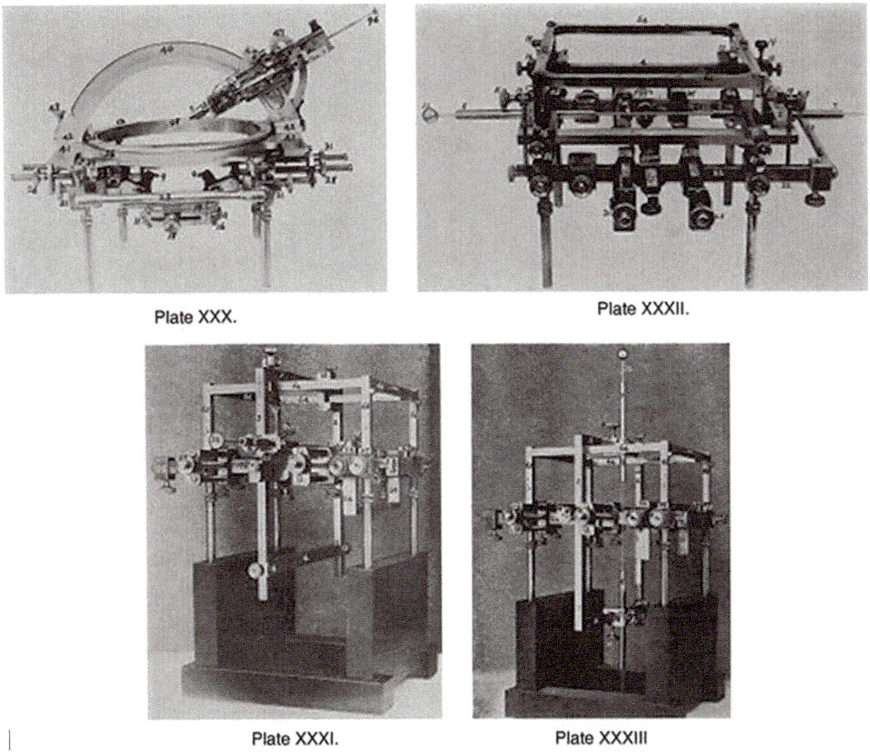

Fig. 4 Horsley and Clarke's stereotaxic frames [12]

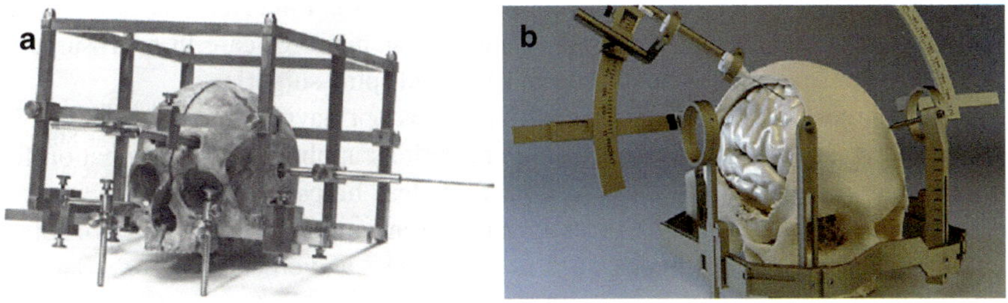

Fig. 5 Stereotaxic frames. (**a**) The first human stereotaxic frame, designed by Mussen [12], (**b**) new version of the stereotaxic frame (https://operativeneurosurgery.com/doku.php?id=stereotactic_biopsy)

In the late 1980s, four different research groups concurrently worked on the registration of patient's physical space to CT images at Dartmouth, Aachen, Tokyo, and Vanderbilt. Their prototypes could dynamically show the tool tip mapped to its corresponding location in images. The Viewing Wand system (ISG Technologies, Canada) was the first frameless neurosurgery navigation device, as shown in Fig. 6. Its mechanical arm with six joints and six degrees of freedom worked as a digitizer and was interfaced to a computer graphics workstation to send the positioning status data [16].

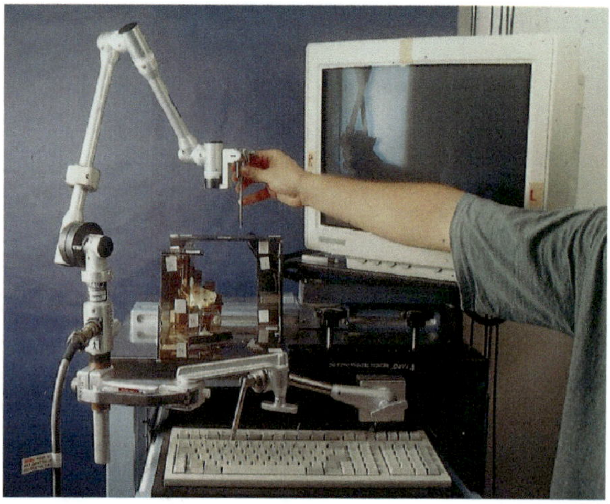

Fig. 6 The ISG Viewing Wand system components as a first navigation system [15]

The articulated arms were relatively heavy with a large inertia. As a result, triangulation systems such as sonic and optical systems as an alternative to arms being considered as physical space localizers. This new insight into the localizers led to the evolution of the registration process in these systems. Therefore, following the debut of the ISG Viewing Wand navigation system, other firms immediately followed suit with a focus on the advanced localizer and registration process, and research into the use of surgical navigation systems swiftly expanded to other anatomical areas. This technique was termed frameless stereotaxic due to the absence of a stereotactic frame. It was later dubbed as the navigation system. Studies have demonstrated that this device improves surgical outcomes, makes surgery less invasive, and reduces the risk of complications and infection. Finally, in the early 2000s, the navigation system was accepted as the gold standard of care in neurosurgery, and it was also growing in popularity in sinus and spine surgeries.

Neurosurgery was the first surgical field to adopt navigation and successfully integrated it into clinical routine. There are various applications of navigation for neurosurgery, including tumor resection, frameless biopsy, screw placement, and stabilization in spine surgery. Currently, navigation supports a broad range of surgical interventions and disciplines, such as ENT, CMF, and others.

Based on the application, we can categorize the navigation systems into the following[1]:

- Neurosurgery navigation systems.
- Orthopedic navigation systems.
- ENT navigation systems.
- Dental and CMF navigation systems.

[1] https://www.medgadget.com/2020/03/surgical-navigation-systems-market-to-reach-usd-1-21-billion-by-2026.html

CMF was one of the surgical specialties that evolved into navigation later in life. Perhaps navigation was first used in the CMF field in the early 1990s [16]. S. Haflfeld and colleagues applied the navigation system to CMF surgery in 1995 and previously by using the Viewing Wand navigation system. They anticipated an increase in surgical quality and a decrease in surgical risks due to the use of computer-assisted simulation and navigation systems. They performed navigation in 40 interventions and reported three cases, including detecting a foreign body, planning of mid-facial osteotomies, and mid-facial and skull base tumor resection. They stated that the accuracy of navigation was approximately 2 mm.

Nowadays, the navigation system is used in a variety of CMF surgical procedures, such as orthognathic and reconstructive surgery, assessment of fractured bone placement during reduction surgery, removal of foreign bodies, tumor resection, temporomandibular joint surgery, dental and craniofacial implantology, and guiding the surgeon in performing precise and sufficient dissection [17, 18].

Multiple firms are now working in the navigation industry. The players in the surgical navigation systems market are 7D Surgical (Canada), Aesculap Implant Systems, Inc. (USA), Amplitude Surgical (France), Augmedics (USA), B. Braun (United Kingdom), Brainlab AG (Germany), Carl Zeiss AG (Germany), ClaroNav (Canada), EPED Inc., Fiagon AG (Germany), GE Health Care (UK), IVS Solutions (Germany), Karl Storz Gmbh & co. kg. (Germany), Mariner Endosurgery Inc. (Canada), Medtronic (Ireland), Navigate Surgical Technologies (Canada), Parsiss (Iran), Scopis (Germany), Stryker Corporation (USA), and UEG Medical Group Ltd. (China) (Table 1).

Table 1 Commercially available navigation systems (the list in alphabetical order)

Company	Legal headquarter	Field of activity
7D Surgical	Toronto, Canada	Neurosurgery, spine
AESCULAP implant systems	Pennsylvania, United States	Orthopedic
Amplitude Surgical	France	Orthopedic
Augmedics	Arlington, United States	Spine
B. Braun	Sheffield, United Kingdom	Orthopedic
Brainlab AG	Munich, Germany	Neurosurgery, ENT and CMF, spine surgery, traumatic interventions
ClaroNav	Toronto, Canada	Dental, ENT, neurosurgery
EPED Inc.	Kaohsiung City, Taiwan	Neurosurgery, ENT, maxillofacial surgery
Fiagon AG	Hennigsdorf, Germany	Neurosurgery, ENT, spine, CMF
GE Health Care	Buckinghamshire, UK	Facial surgery
IVS Solutions	Chemnitz, Germany	CMF
Karl Storz Gmbh & co. kg.	Tuttlingen, Germany	ENT, skull base surgery
Mariner Endosurgery Inc	Canada	Endo-surgery
Medtronic	Dublin, Ireland	ENT, neurosurgery and spine

(continued)

Table 1 (continued)

Company	Legal headquarter	Field of activity
Navigate Surgical Technologies	Vancouver, Canada	Dental
Parsiss	Tehran, Iran	Neurosurgery, ENT, spine, CMF
Scopis	Berlin, Germany	ENT, maxillofacial, neurosurgery, spine
Stryker Corporation	Kalamazoo, Michigan, United States	Neurosurgery, spinal surgery, ENT and orthopedic, CMF
UEG Medical Group Ltd	Shanghai, China	CMF

In general, the three major players in this market are Medtronic Plc., Stryker Corporation, and Brainlab.[2] Among these companies, 3dsystems, Brainlab, Carl Zeiss AG, EPED, Fiagon AG, GE Health Care, IVS Solutions, Parsiss, Stryker, and UEG medical are active in the field of CMF, as shown in Table 2. Also, two examples of commercial surgical navigations being used in the CMF field have been shown in Fig. 7.

After getting acquainted with a short history of navigation systems, the following sections will discuss the surgical navigation principle, which includes imaging modalities as an integral part of the navigation system, tracking systems, and registration processes, along with the fundamental concept, error analysis, and registration accuracy improvement, as well as the limitations, improvement, and future of navigation systems.

2 Principal of Navigation Systems

Typically, navigated surgery is divided into three main stages: imaging, tracking, and registration. As shown in Fig. 8, the initial step should be to obtain diagnostic images of the patient prior to surgery and upload them to navigation systems, and then anatomical landmarks are selected determined on the image. Different imaging modalities such as CT and cone-beam computed tomography (CBCT) which could be used in this part will be reviewed in Sect. 2.1. In the second stage, navigation tool is tracked using tracking system. Various tracking systems considering all of the advantages and disadvantages, which are used to track surgical tools, will be discussed in Sect. 2.2 in detail. Finally, the preoperative image should be registered with the patient's position in a real-time process using the registration techniques outlined in Sect. 2.3. As a result, the preoperative dataset displayed on the navigation screen corresponds to the patient's real-time and spatial position on the surgical table.

[2] https://www.alliedmarketresearch.com/surgical-navigation-systems-market

Table 2 The list of companies that are active in the production of navigation systems and software in the CMF field (the list in alphabetical order)

Company	Products name	Field of activity
3dsystems	VSP Orthognathics, VSP Reconstruction, VSP Cranial, VSP Distraction, VSP Trauma, and Jaw in a Day	CMF surgical planning
Brainlab	Vector Vision, Digital CMF Surgery	CMF surgery, surgical planning, mixed reality viewing, surgical navigation
Carl Zeiss AG	Surgical Segment Navigator (SSN)	Bone segment navigation, osteotomy, orthognathic surgery [19]
EPED	RETINA	Craniofacial, plastic surgery, oral and maxillofacial surgery, and other types of minimally invasive surgical applications
Fiagon AG	Fiagon ENT Navigation System	CMF surgery, ENT
GE Health Care	Instatrak	Facial surgery
IVS Solutions	VoNaviX, Voxim	Craniomaxillofacial surgery
Parsiss	Compo+	Orthognathic surgery, reconstruction surgery, TMJ surgery, zygomatic arch surgery, oral-maxillofacial trauma surgery, etc.
Stryker	Stryker Navigation System, working in collaboration with 3D Systems provided virtual surgery planning: VSP® solutions, VSP® Cranial, VSP® Reconstruction, VSP® Orthognathic	Aesthetics, orthognathic, reconstruction, trauma
UEG medical	AccuNavi-A navigation system	Plastic reconstructive surgery, TMJ surgery, orthognathic surgery, oral-maxillofacial injury surgery, temporal surgery with complex structure, restoration surgery of eye socket and midface, zygomatic arch surgery, bone grafts, reshaping surgery, etc.

Imaging

Visualization of interesting regions in preoperative images during the surgical process is an essential requirement for the navigation system. In other words, the fundamental basis of navigation systems is image. The surgeon navigates the surgical tool and visualizes it on preoperative images, which are provided using a wide range of imaging techniques; all of them are associated with specific advantages and disadvantages. There is no unique imaging modality that is exclusively used in navigation systems, so the selection of preoperative images is dependent on a specific application. There are two broad categories of imaging modalities: structural and functional imaging. Structural imaging, which includes magnetic resonance imaging (MRI), CT, and ultrasound, etc., is a term that refers to techniques for

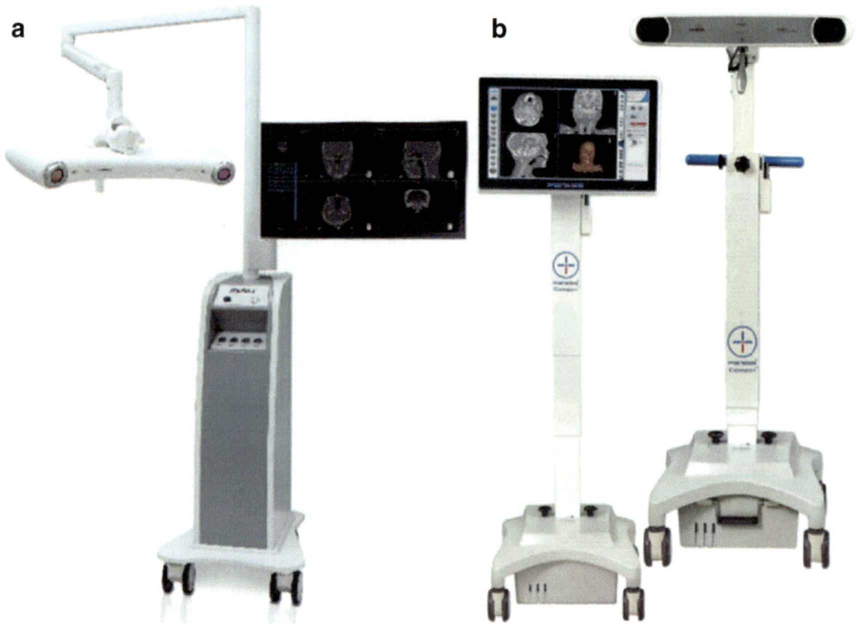

Fig. 7 Two commercial surgical navigations are used in CMF field. (**a**) RETINA (EPED INC.) is a navigation system for neurosurgery, ENT, plastic surgery, oral and maxillofacial surgery (https://www.epedmed.com/retina), (**b**) Compo+ (PARSISS. Co), a comprehensive and high-performance surgical navigation system for neurosurgery and ENT, spine, and maxillofacial surgeries (https://www. PARSISS.com/products/Compo)

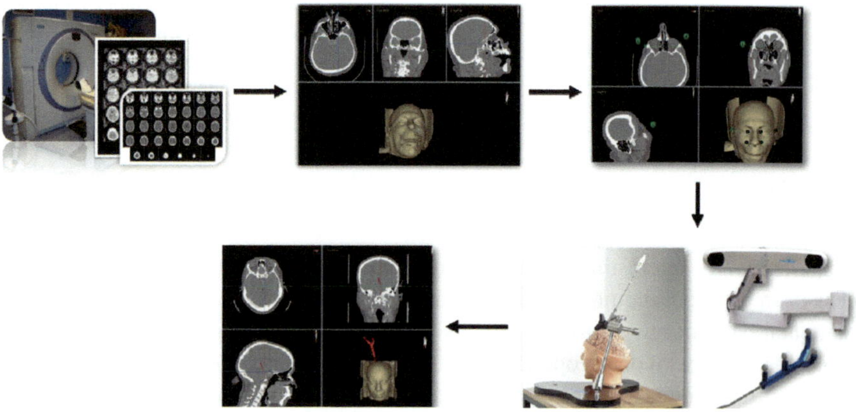

Fig. 8 Workflow of navigation

visualizing and analyzing anatomical structures. In contrast to structural imaging, functional imaging, including positron emission tomography (PET), functional MRI (fMRI), and diffusion tensor imaging (DTI), is applied to detect or measure

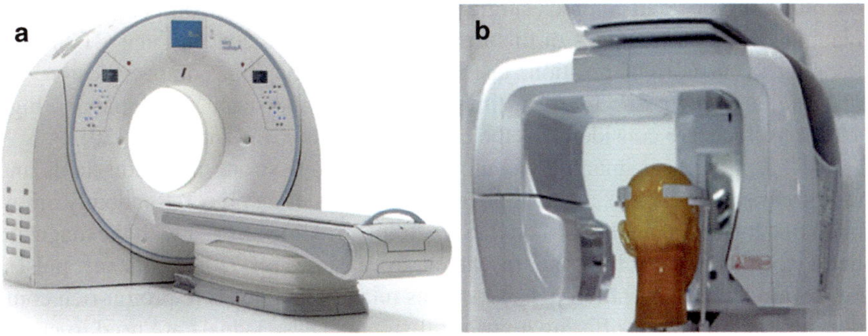

Fig. 9 (**a**) Modern CT scanner (https://my.medical.canon/products/computed-tomography), (**b**) CBCT system [20]

changes in metabolism, blood flow, regional chemical composition, and absorption. The following sections address the most major imaging modalities used in navigation systems and their applications in the CMF area.

CT as one of the most widely used diagnostic imaging modalities is very effective in various applications, including cancer imaging, cardiovascular disease, abdomen imaging, internal injuries and angiography, infection, treatment plans and procedures for biopsies, surgeries, and radiation therapy. CT scanners (Fig. 9a) calculate X-ray attenuation in different tissues of the body using a rotating geometry X-ray tube and an array of detectors positioned on the gantry. This modality is capable of producing high-resolution images and accurately representing the bone tissue and bony structures. However, along with these benefits, there are several disadvantages, such as high dose to the patient, high cost, partial volume effect, and imaging in the supine position, which may result in anatomical changes [21].

The images generated using conventional X-rays and CT imaging are confined to a 2D representation of a 3D anatomy. Whereas CBCT is a special type of conventional CT that provides 3D anatomical information about the patient (Fig. 9b). Therefore, a CBCT can provide volumetric information about the various organs, such as the oral and maxillofacial regions, teeth, ears, nose, and throat. CBCT uses a conical or pyramidal shaped X-ray to produce a 3D image of anatomy.[3] CBCT is a valuable imaging technique in dentistry and CMF surgery. Attilio Tacconi and Piero Mozzo developed the first CBCT system for maxillofacial applications in 1995, which was manufactured by QR Inc. [22]. The total radiation doses from dental CBCT exams are lower than conventional CT and have a relatively better spatial resolution. Today, dental CBCT has various clinical applications, including skeletal and dental imaging, implant planning, orthognathic surgical planning, evaluation of the jaws and face for surgery planning, cleft palate assessment, endodontic diagnosis, and diagnosis of facial and dental trauma, reconstruction surgery,

[3] https://www.fda.gov/radiation-emitting-products/medical-x-ray-imaging/dental-cone-beam-computed-tomography

oncology surgery, and complex surgical procedures that require proper preoperative planning. Other advantages of this imaging compared to conventional CT include imaging in an upright position, fast and accurate imaging, compact design, 3D imaging, and low cost. However, limited scan field and scanned volume and high scatter artifacts are considered as the disadvantages of CBCT imaging [20].

MRI is a medical imaging technique that employs strong magnetic fields and radiofrequency waves to create high-contrast images of an object. Randomly orientated free hydrogen nuclei (protons) in the object become aligned with the magnetic field. Protons are excited and resonated by a series of radiofrequency pulses. Following the RF excitation pulses, protons relax, which leads to proton-rich components such as water offering a powerful signal. These signals are used to create MRI images. MRI can reveal finer details than CT, particularly in tumors and soft tissue due to their water content level. However, because bony structures contain little water, MRI is unable to reflect them adequately. The advantages of MRI include the non-ionizing nature of the image capturing and the ability to demonstrate soft tissue with high contrast. The downsides of MR imaging include the expense, time of examination, and inability to demonstrate the bony structures. MRI is the gold standard for determining the disc–condyle relationship, evaluating abnormalities in the temporal mandibular joint and masticatory muscles, as well as the presentation of ligaments and cartilaginous discs is MRI [23].

Ultrasound (US), alternatively referred to as sonography, creates an image by utilizing ultrasonic waves, sound waves with frequencies higher than the upper audible limit of human hearing, and their echoes from within the body. It is a non-ionizing, noninvasive, and low-cost imaging modality that provides real-time images. The disadvantages of the US include limited contrast and image quality. Ultrasound imaging is also used in the CMF area in applications such as periodontal assessment tool pocket depth, tissue thickness, histological change, calculus, and determination of gingival thickness.

As we mentioned, in contrast to structural imaging, functional imaging measures changes in metabolism. PET is one of these imaging modalities that examines the function and metabolism of tissue or organs by using radioactive substances (radiotracers). The commonly used positron-emitting substances are ^{18}F, ^{11}C, ^{15}O, ^{13}N, ^{68}Ga, and ^{82}Rb. In the positron annihilation process, it generates two anti-parallel 511 Kev photons that are detected by detectors to create an image. PET has a lot of applications in CMF, such as tumor detection, staging, treatment planning, and evaluation of tumor recurrence and follow-up controls. DTI and fMRI are specific MRI techniques. The fMRI indirectly measures brain activity (local cerebral blood flow), and DTI is a technique used to detect how water passes through the white matter tracts of the brain.

Finally, the advantages and disadvantages of various structural and functional imaging modalities with their applications in the CMF field are compared in Table 3.

Table 3 Advantages and disadvantages of different structural and functional imaging

Modality	Advantages	Disadvantages	Application in CMF
CT	High resolution Visualization of bone tissue and bone structure	High patient dose Cost Partial volume effect Imaging in the supine position	Diagnostic and surgical planning of CMF [21]
CBCT	Imaging in an upright position Fast, compact, and low dose High resolution and accurate 3D imaging Low cost	Limited scan field High scatter artifacts	Skeletal and dental imaging Diagnostic and surgical planning of CMF
MRI	Nonionizing High contrast Soft tissue imaging	Cost Exam duration Inability to display bony structures	Temporomandibular joint Masticatory muscles Condylar erosion and effusion Ligament and cartilaginous disc [24]
Ultrasound	Nonionizing Noninvasive Inexpensive Real-time	Low contrast Low quality Image deformation	Periodontal assessment tool Pocket depth, attachment level, tissue thickness, histological change, calculus, determination of gingival thickness [25, 26]
PET	Providing metabolic and functional information	Patient dose Expensive Motion artifacts	Tumor detection and staging Treatment planning, evaluation of tumor recurrence Follow-up controls [27]

Imaging Artifacts

Regardless of the relative merits and demerits of each imaging modality, one of the major factors affecting the accuracy of the navigation system is the quality of the preoperative images, which is affected by image artifacts. Artifacts are just one of the several factors that might degrade the quality of medical imaging data. An artifact is an artificial feature in an image that does not exist in the original object, but it makes damages to diagnosis and interpretation of images. Therefore, prior to using images for diagnosis or treatment, it is required to evaluate the images and, if necessary, minimize artifacts using image processing techniques and, in certain situations, retake images.

Metal artifacts, patient motion artifacts, aliasing artifacts, beam hardening artifacts, ring artifacts, and partial volume effect are all described in the literature as common artifacts across almost all medical imaging modalities. Here, we focus on the widespread artifacts in CT and CBCT modalities, which are the most commonly used imaging techniques in CMF filed.

Metal artifacts occur when an object contains highly absorbing material, such as amalgam fillings, implants, crowns, or bridges. When X-rays are incident on these dense materials, the image quality degrades accompanied by streak artifacts in the image. It appears as a series of white and black lines [28] (Fig. 10a), and the presence of a metallic item obscures the area of interest.

Patient motion artifacts manifest as blurred or streaked lines in a reconstructed image and are frequently visible as double contours or ghost images [28]. This characteristic precludes the image from being used for diagnosis or treatment planning, and the imaging must be redone (Fig. 10b).

Aliasing artifacts are created by cone-beam divergence-induced under-sampling. Aliasing becomes visible in the image as fine striations diverge from the center to the perimeter. As shown in Fig. 10c, fine striations diverge from the center to the perimeter, indicating aliasing.

The polychromatic nature of the X-ray causes *beam hardening artifacts*. When low-energy rays pass through a higher-attenuating object, they are absorbed [34]. As a consequence, the average beam energy increases (hardens). The artifact causes dark streaks in the reconstructed image (Fig. 10d) [35].

Defective or un-calibrated detectors cause the *ring artifact*. Ring artifacts appear as concentric rings in the reconstructed image centered on the axis of rotation (Fig. 10e) [35].

Partial volume effect or partial volume averaging occurs when an off-center dense object protrudes partially into the X-ray beam. This phenomenon occurs when the voxel size is larger than the spatial resolution of the object to be captured. For example, a partial volume effect appears when surfaces change rapidly in the z-direction, e.g., temporal bone (Fig. 10f). This artifact can be reduced by selecting the smallest image voxel size.

Overall, the artifacts lead to inaccurate diagnosis and misinterpretations and should be compensated. Reduction of reconstructed image quality due to the presence of artifacts leads to inaccurate patient-to-image registration in navigation systems.

Tracking Systems

Object tracking is an integral part of the context of interventional medicine, particularly in the field of IGS. Tracking systems through interaction with images obtained before operations (e.g., tomographic images) offer continual tracking of tools, accurate targeting, reduction of medical procedure time, and finally, reducing the patient's pain through minimally invasive approaches. In IGS systems, preoperative images are carefully assessed to determine the Region of Interest (ROI) and plan for surgery. To perform real-time intraoperative tracking of surgical tools, preoperative images must be registered with the patient's physical space. Various techniques have been introduced for image-to-patient registration in the literature [36] that will be discussed more in detail in Sect. 2.3. With corresponding preoperative

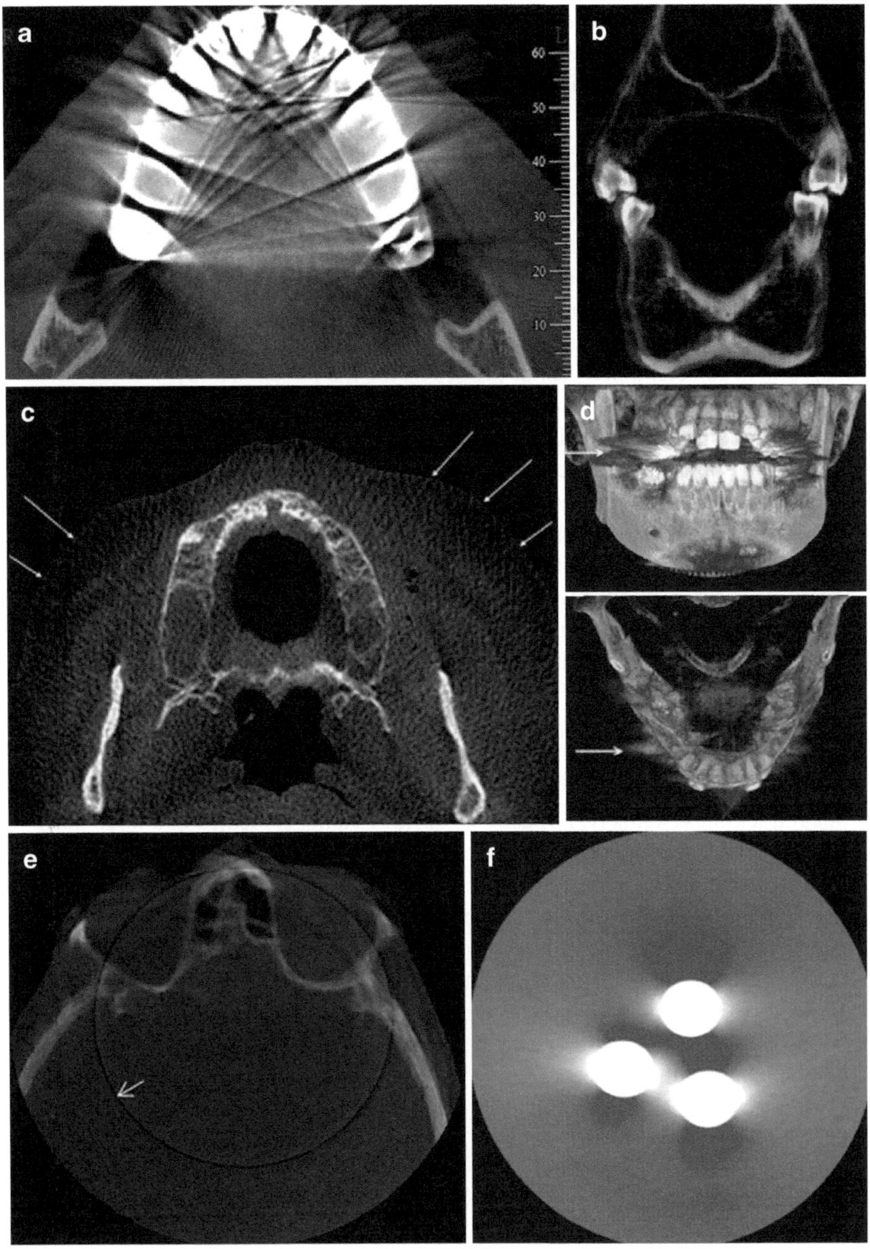

Fig. 10 Imaging artifacts. (**a**) CBCT image of the dental contains a metal artifact. The silver amalgam crowns cause streak artifacts that appear as white and black lines [29], (**b**) Bilateral motion artifacts in the upper and lower jaws. The artifacts are oriented buccolingually [28], (**c**) Typical aliasing patterns on CBCT data are indicated by the arrows [30], (**d**) Beam hardening effect on 3D image (arrows) [31], (**e**) A ring artifact created by a defective detector element [32], (**f**) Partial volume artifact which appears in the reconstructed image obtained with the rods partially intruded into the width of the section [33]

information of the patient to the intraoperative surgical anatomy, the pose of the navigating tool can be visualized in the preoperative imaging data. The IGS system's accuracy is directly related to the tracking techniques used in navigation systems.

Optical tracking systems (OTS) and electromagnetic tracking (EMT) systems are the most promising navigation systems for IGS applications. A typical OTS uses cameras for stereo-photogrammetric localization of tools. The pose of the tools in the camera's working space is being tracked based on stereo visualization techniques. The primary advantage of this system is attributed to high accuracy measurements of surgical instruments and its robustness to environmental distortions [37]. However, light blocking is the main disadvantage of OTS when the intervention requires catheters, needles, or probes inside the patient's body.

In contrast, EMT systems provide advantages like fast-tracking without line-of-sight restrictions that enable instruments to move freely without any need to interfere with the source of the tracking system [38]. But, compared with OTS, they have less precision and are highly prone to distortion from metallic or ferromagnetic objects inside their working space in the operating room [39]. The main components of an OTS and an EMT system and their integration into a generic surgical scenario are shown in Fig. 11. A few examples of IGS systems regarding their applications in medicine are summarized in Table 4. In the following subsection, the two tracking systems will be discussed in detail.

Optical Tracking Systems

Optical tracking systems (OTS) use two or three cameras located in a fixed place to provide visual information from tracked tools. OTS are divided into video-metric and near-infrared (IR) tracking systems, which are tuned for ambient and IR light, retrospectively. Video-metric systems track a geometric printed pattern, using image processing and data fitting approaches, on markers. Tracking objects are equipped with two or three markers with a checkered pattern, which rectangles cross in "XPoints" [53]. Calibrated video cameras detect the position and orientation of tracking objects in 3D by using at least three vectors (facets) formed by connecting XPoints. One of the commercially available video-metric systems is ClaroNav (Toronto, Ontario, Canada) (Fig. 12). The marker tracking accuracy in these systems is 0.2 mm [54].

The cameras in IR tracking systems are two planar or three CCD cameras equipped with IR passing filters and a circular arrangement of IR LEDs around the lens, so IR systems are not influenced by ambient light. In these systems, markers are fixed in a rigid alignment on the navigating tool and, based on transmitting or reflecting light, are divided into active or passive markers. Active markers are infrared-emitting diodes that need a cable attached to them, while wireless passive markers are typically retro-reflective spheres and are more widely used in operating rooms (see Fig. 13). The 3D location of the tracking object is determined based on

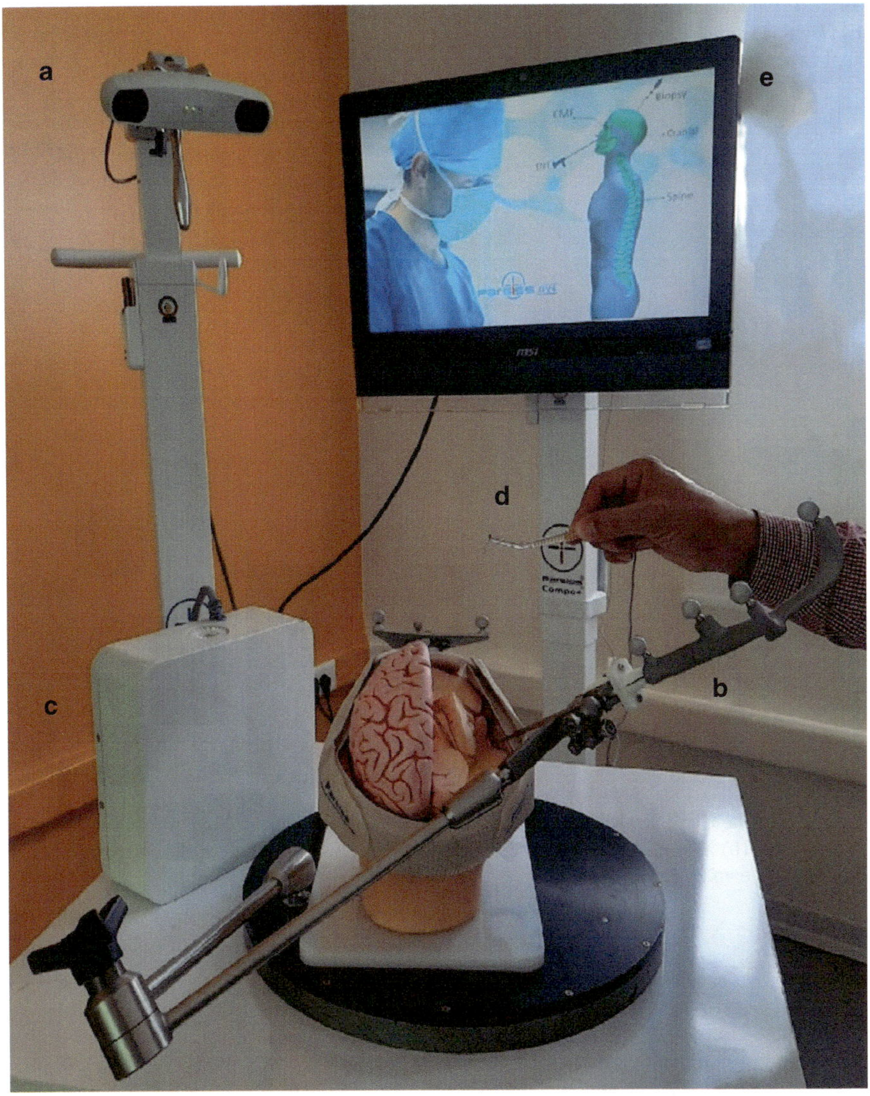

Fig. 11 The main components of optical and electromagnetic tracking systems are presented. OTS contains an optical camera (**a**) and an optical tool (**b**). EMT system includes a field generator (**c**), an electromagnetic tool (**d**), and a workstation (**e**)

triangulation and known geometrical configuration of markers and distance between CCD cameras [43].

The main commercially available optical trackers for medical applications are fusionTrack (Atracsys Inc., Puidoux, Switzerland) and Polaris (NDI Inc., Ontario, Canada) (see Fig. 14).

Table 4 Optical and EMT-guided surgery systems application in medicine

	Clinical applications
Optical-based	Cranial and spinal [5, 40] Neurosurgery [41] Orthopedic [42] ENT [43] Dental implant placement [44] Biopsy procedure [45] Laparoscopy [46]
EMT-based	Oral and maxillofacial [47] Endoscopy [48] Bronchoscopy [49] ENT [50] Neurosurgery [51] Catheter tracking [52]

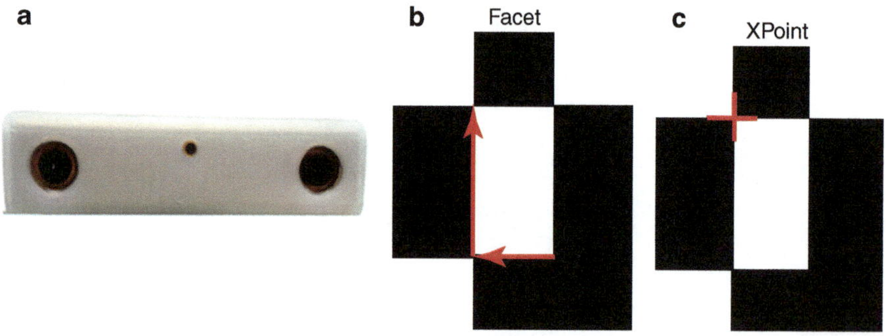

Fig. 12 (**a**) The ClaroNav Micron Tracker includes two digital cameras and ambient visible light in the center. (**b**) X-point is defined as the black–white intersection point. (**c**) Two vectors describe a facet are shown by red arrows

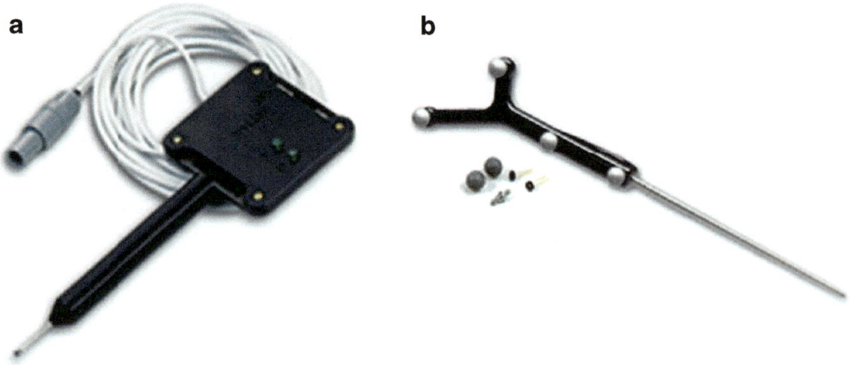

Fig. 13 Examples of optical tracking tools. (**a**) A tool with active markers, (**b**) a tool with passive sphere markers

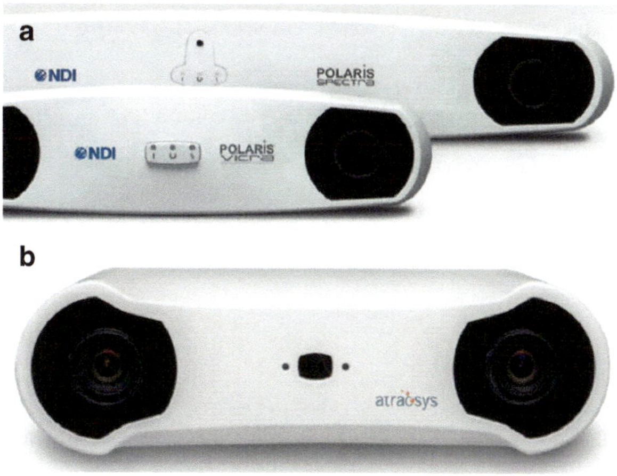

Fig. 14 Commonly employed optical tracking systems. (**a**) Polaris Spectra and Polaris Vicra from NDI (https://www.ndigital.com/), (**b**) fusionTrack from Atracsys (https://www.atracsys-measurement.com/)

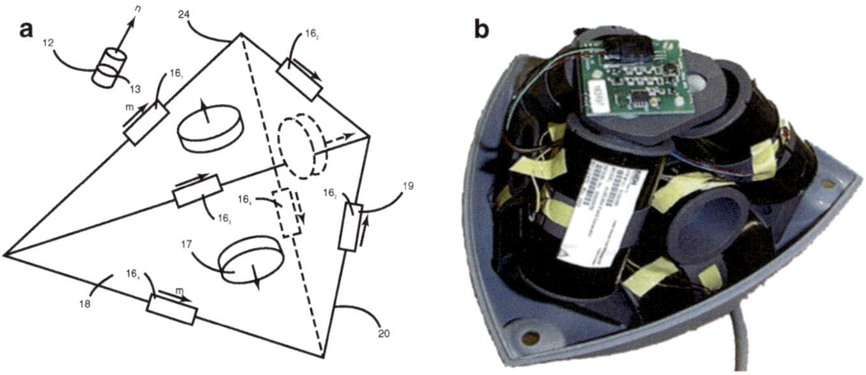

Fig. 15 An example of internal coil configuration of Northern Digital, Inc's (NDI's) Aurora EMF first generation. (**a**) Internal coil configuration. Photograph courtesy of Northern Digital Inc. (**b**) Photograph of the corresponding coils in an open NDI FG

A clear line-of-sight is required between the camera and the markers. Also, any infrared light from other sources must be covered. Hence, surgical tools outside the body can be tracked by OTS, and they are not suitable for tracking flexible tools (like endoscopes) because a fixed relationship between the tool's tip and the tracker is needed [55]. Nevertheless, higher accuracy and reliability (e.g., accuracy of 0.25 m with an NDI Polaris Spectra optical tracker system and an accuracy of 0.09 m up to 2 m with a fusionTrack 500 system) and larger working volume (e.g., a pyramidal ($2400 \times 1566 \times 1312$ mm^3) or extended pyramidal ($3000 \times 1856 \times 1470$ mm^3) with NDI Polaris Spectra optical tracker systems) make them suitable for many surgical applications [55]. Additionally, OTS do not suffer from interference from electromagnetic objects or other IR devices.

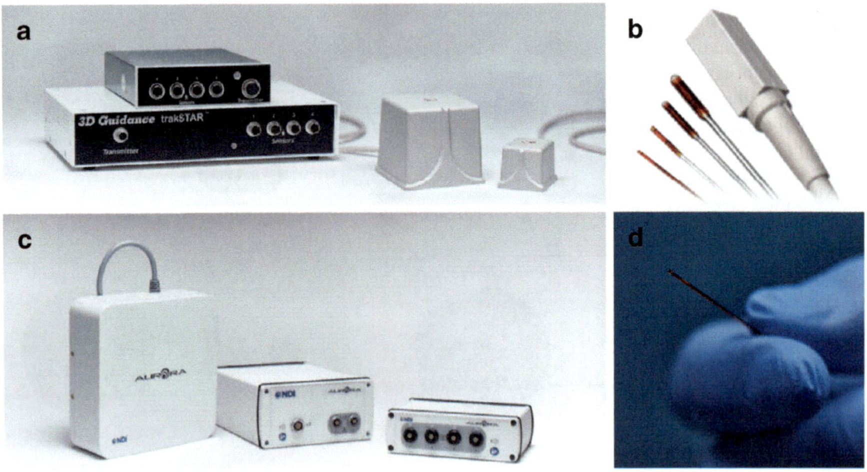

Fig. 16 Examples of field generators and sensors for EM tracking. Photograph courtesy of Northern Digital Inc. (NDI) and Ascension Technology Corporation. (**a**) Example of Ascension tracking system field generator, control unit, and sensor interface unit, (**b**) Different sensors for the Ascension tracking system, (**c**) Example of NDI tracking system field generator, control unit, and sensor interface unit, (**d**) 6DOF sensor for the NDI Aurora

EMT Systems

Electromagnetic tracking (EMT) systems without line-of-sight restrictions have been introduced to medical applications as a potential method for real-time navigation of medical instruments with respect to the patient's anatomy [49]. They are widely applied in a diversity of fields, especially during endoscopy, tumor therapy, gene therapy, neurosurgery, cardiology, catheter tracking, and 3D ultrasound [56].

EMT systems are based on the localization of six degrees of freedom (DOF) sensors within a magnetic field generator, created by field transmitters. To obtain six DOF, a magnetic field transmitter with three orthogonal coils is coupled to a receiver (sensor) with three coils via driving circuits. An example of an EMT system FG is shown in Fig. 15. A sequential pulse flows through the coils and induces a voltage in the electromagnetic (EM) sensor coils embedded in the magnetic field. The EM system can calculate the sensor's position by comparing the strength of the received signals and sent pulses and comparing them with one another to determine the orientation.

Several EMT systems have been developed commercially. Two examples of available systems for medical purposes are Ascension Technology (Burlington, VT, USA) with a position accuracy of 1.4 mm and an orientation accuracy of 0.5° for trakSTAR systems in a cubic working volume of $160 \times 160 \times 160$ mm^3 and Northern Digital (NDI) Inc. (Waterloo, ON, Canada) with a position accuracy of 0.48 mm and an orientation accuracy of 0.30° in a cubic working volume of $500 \times 500 \times 500$ mm^3 [38] (Fig. 16).

Unfortunately, EMT systems are prone to errors as a result of magnetic field distortions caused by ferromagnetic materials and eddy currents. These distortions are referred to as systematic errors [57]. Certain types of EMT systems eliminate eddy currents by employing pulsed quasi-static DC fields. However, ferromagnetic materials according to their permeability and the frequency of the electromagnetic field generator will affect the tracking accuracy of both AC and DC systems. The other source of errors is caused by sensor movement and changes in external electromagnetic fields; these are referred to as dynamic errors.

While it is possible to compensate for systematic errors via calibration at the system level, dynamic effects, particularly in environments like operating rooms, are probably the most concerning drawback. One way to overcome static errors in EMT systems is to find mismatches between actual positions and reported positions by the EMT system. Tracker calibration is the term used to describe this procedure. The distortion map can be described as different techniques, such as 3D interpolation, shape function mapping, high-order polynomial fit, or neural networks. Afterward, this mapping can be employed intraoperatively to compensate for the unwanted static distortion. However, calibration is a time-consuming procedure because the sensor needs to be placed in different known positions in the workspace. Furthermore, the distortion map is valid as long as the environment stays static. Sensor positioning can be done manually on a calibration phantom or automatically by using a robotic arm that acquires a higher number of data points. A few studies have worked on dynamical error reduction approaches. The proposed methods try to use a set of EM sensors and the motion model of the object to find the distortion map and accurate object's position in a real-time procedure [58, 59].

Registration

One of the most fundamental prerequisites and critical steps in navigation systems is the image registration procedure. Image registration is the process of determining a spatial transformation that overlays two or more images of the same scene which are obtained at different times, from different viewpoints, or with different imaging sensors [60]. Based on this definition, there are various applications for image registration, including diagnosis, such as combining data from multiple imaging modalities to acquire more information, studying disease progressions, such as tracking and monitoring changes in size, shape, position, or intensity of the particular target over time, image-guided surgeries and radiotherapies, such as relating preoperative images and surgical plans, patient comparison, or atlas construction, such as relating one individual's anatomy to a standardized atlas. An example of the application of image registration in image-guided surgery can be seen in Fig. 17, which finds corresponding points in preoperative data (MRI and CT) and intraoperative space.

The ultimate goal of image registration is to optimize transformation (T), which aligns a target or moving image to a source or fixed image as shown in Fig. 18. In

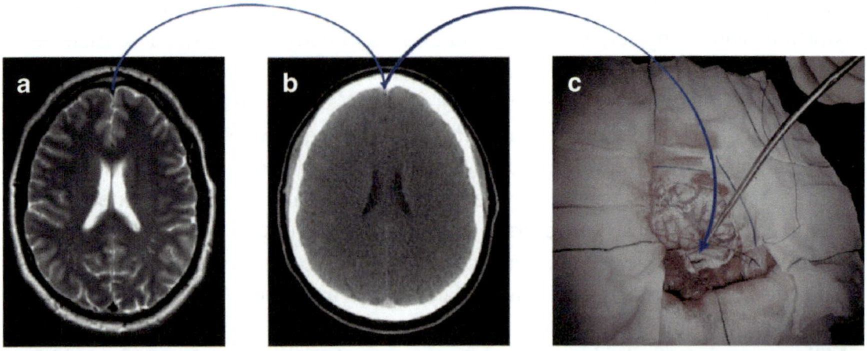

Fig. 17 An example of image registration in image-guided surgery. (**a**) Preoperative MRI, and (**b**) preoperative CT of patient, (**c**) intraoperative space. The blue arrows indicate corresponding points in three spaces

Fig. 18 Schematic of the image registration procedure

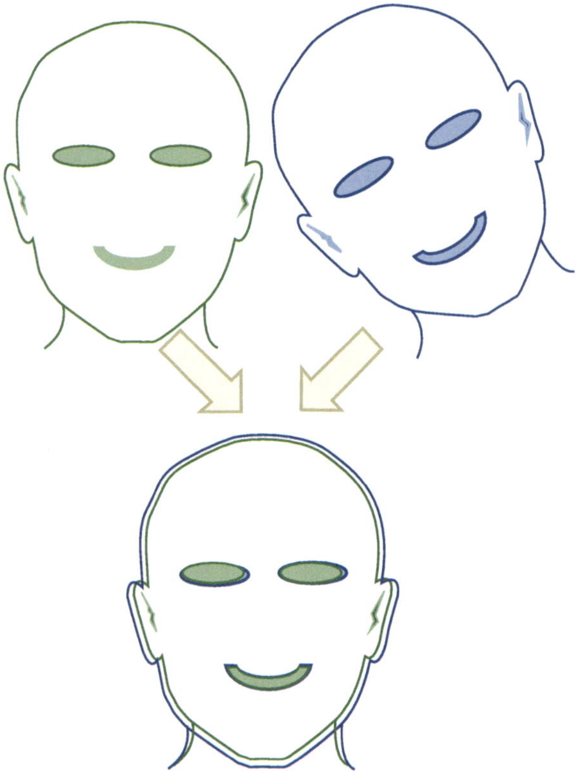

fact, the image registration procedure includes three main steps: (1) determination of the transformation between the source image and the target image, (2) measuring the similarity measure, and (3) optimizing the transformation [61].

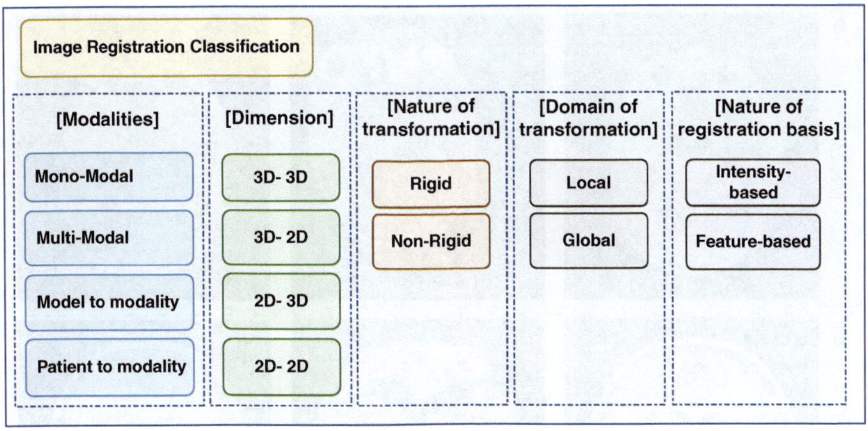

Fig. 19 Image registration classification based on different basic criteria

There are different classifications for registration approaches based on a variety of characteristics, the most critical of which are as follows: *modalities involved, dimension, nature of transformation, domain of transformation, and nature of registration basis*, as we have shown in Fig. 19.

Registration methods are categorized into four categories based on the *modalities* involved: mono-modal, multi-modal, model to modality, and patient to modality. Mono-modal registration, which aligns images of the same modality to one another, can be applied to the same patients to monitor and quantify disease progression over time (Fig. 20a), or to separate patients for purposes such as atlas construction and investigation of subject variability.

Multi-modal registration, which aligns images of different modalities, is typically used for two main purposes: combining information obtained from disparate modalities, such as MRI-PET registration (Fig. 20b), and calculating organ deformations. Also, there is a model to modality registration, which aligns models (often 3D models) obtained from any organ or lesion with their corresponding image (Fig. 20c). Finally, patient to modality registration, which is employed exclusively in IGS procedures, accurately aligns the patient's location with preoperative images such as CT and MRI.

According to the *dimensions* involved, registration approaches could be classified into 3D-3D, 3D-2D, 2D-3D, and 2D-2D registration, which are referred to volume-to-volume, volume-to-slice, slice-to-volume, and slice-to-slice registration, respectively. For example, in the third case (2D-3D or slice-to-volume registration), each value of a 2D slice of modalities such as ultrasound or MRI could be registered into a corresponding value in a 3D image, space, or model. In the same way, for 3D-3D registration, each value or position in a 3D image, space, or model could be registered into its corresponding position in another 3D image, space, or model.

Also, registration approaches could be applied based on the *domain of transformation*; locally on subsections of the image or globally on the whole image.

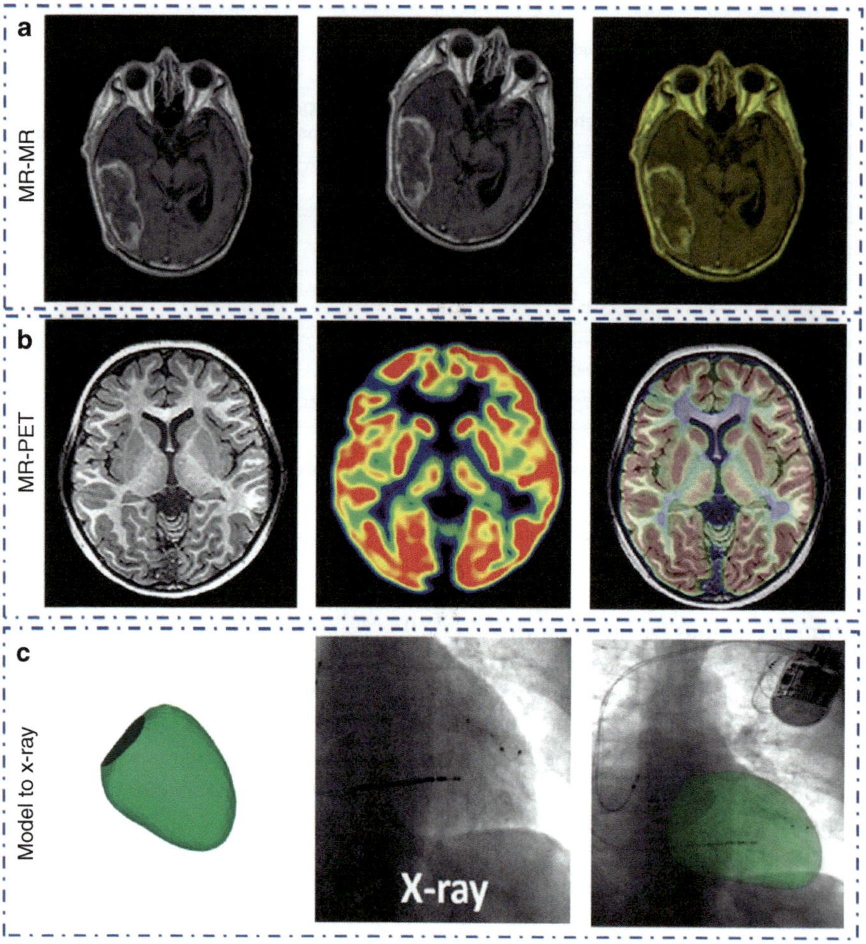

Fig. 20 Example of registration classification based on modalities involved. (**a**) Mono-modal: MRI-MR [62], (**b**) Multi-modal: MRI-PET, (**c**) Model-modality: 3D model to X-ray [63]

According to the *nature of transformations*, registration methods could be classified into rigid and non-rigid transformations. The rigid transformation as a geometric transformation preserves the Euclidean distance between every pair of points and therefore keeps the shape and size of the object. It includes transformations, rotations, reflections, or any combination of them. In contrast, the non-rigid transformation is an unpredictable and nonlinear transformation.

The ultimate goal of image registration in navigation systems is to map preoperative images to patient coordinate systems during surgery. In other words, the preoperative image of the patient should be aligned perfectly with the intraoperative position of the patient. Therefore, the image registration procedure in navigation could be considered a 3D-3D modality-to-patient, rigid, and global problem.

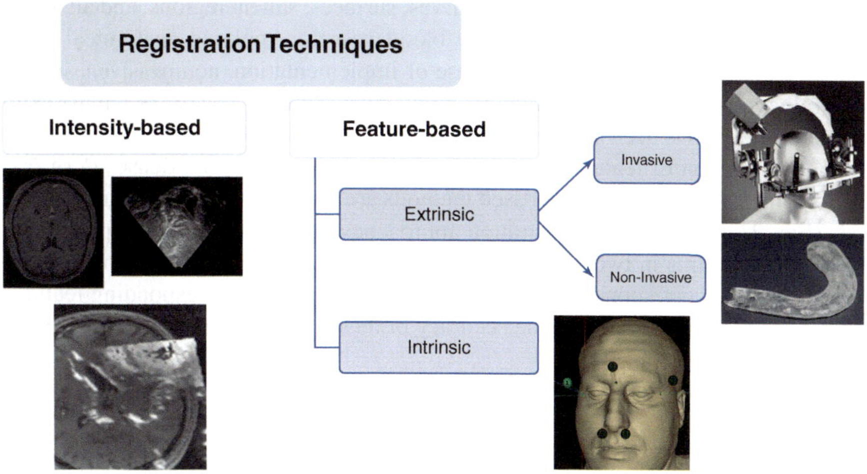

Fig. 21 Classification of registration techniques, including intensity-based registration and feature-based registration. Features could be extrinsic (invasive or noninvasive) or intrinsic

Regardless of dimensions, domain, transform, and modalities, registration techniques could be classified into two main categories based on the *nature of registration*, including intensity-based and feature-based registration techniques, as we have shown in Fig. 21.

Intensity-based registration algorithms are applied over pixels or voxels of images using similarity measures such as mutual information, correlation ratio, or sum square differences to align the pixels in one image into corresponding pixels in another image [61]. However, in the intensity-based methods, due to the different nature of the two imaging modalities (different scale, resolution, etc.), proposing a proper similarity measure could be a challenging task, particularly in multimodal image registration [64]. Moreover, these approaches are predicated on the premise that the pixel/voxel intensities of the two images are related. It is while defining specific relationships across multiple modalities is a difficult undertaking. Additionally, because intensity-based registration algorithms typically make use of every pixel's information, they are frequently time-consuming procedures. Feature-based registration techniques find correspondences between features that are available in either images or spaces. Features that are used during the registration procedures could be classified into *intrinsic* and *extrinsic* features. Extrinsic features are usually markers attached to the organ surface, skin, and bones. These markers could be attached to patients *invasively*, such as stereotactic frames and screw markers, or *noninvasively*, such as dental adapters, skin markers, and frames. Using extrinsic features leads to fast and accurate registration without needing any complex optimization. It is notable that invasive markers have better accuracy in comparison with noninvasive markers. However, markers should be designed and manufactured before starting the procedure. On the other hand, intrinsic features, which are also known as *anatomical features*, are extracted based on the locations or orientation of corners, boundaries, curves, surfaces, salient regions, and also anatomical structures such as tumors and blood vessels. Applying anatomical landmarks is more common due to their ease of implementation, noninvasiveness, and naturalness. An example of anatomical points placed on the face of the Parsiss skull phantom (PSP) has been shown in Fig. 22 [65].

The extraction of features transforms grayscale images into a dense set of discrete points. Therefore, feature-based methods are also known as point-based methods (Fig. 23). Point-based registration approaches iteratively find correspondences between the points in two spaces and then estimate the transformation parameters based on these correspondences. However, extraction of the corresponding features is an issue that directly affects the accuracy of these methods, especially in two different modalities [66].

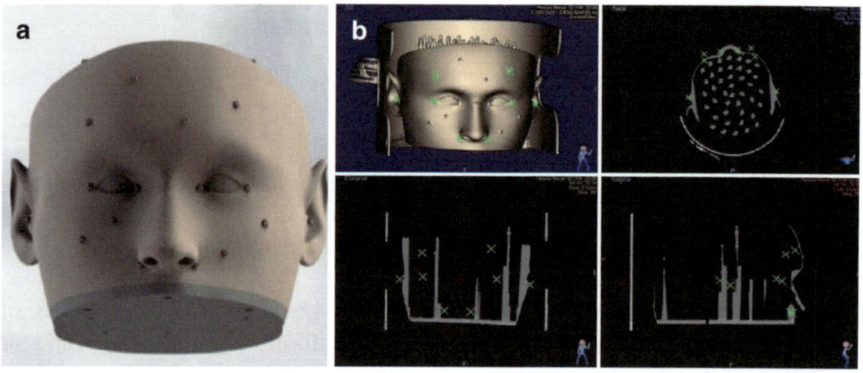

Fig. 22 (**a**) An example of anatomical points placed on the face at PSP, (**b**) selecting the landmarks on the 3D reconstructed image of PSP in three views of axial, coronal, and sagittal [65]

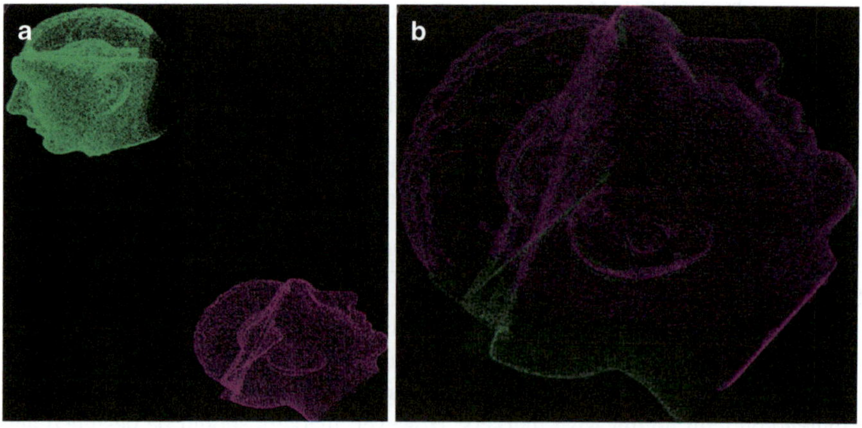

Fig. 23 3D registration of phantom data, (**a**) 3D point cloud of source (green) and target (purple) data, (**b**) 3D registration of two-point sets

In commercial navigation systems, point-based registration methods are broadly adopted and mostly used in existing navigation systems. The iterative closest point (ICP) algorithm, introduced by Besl and McKay [67], is the most popular method for point set registration among others due to its simplicity and low computational complexity [68]. The ICP algorithm in the first step assigns correspondences between the two cloud points based on the closest Euclidean distance criterion and then finds the least-squares rigid transformation relating the two-point sets. The ICP iteratively repeats these two steps to converge on the desired transformation. If the exact correspondence between the two data sets could be known, then the exact translation and rotation could be found. Despite the high-speed convergence of the ICP algorithm, it may converge toward local minima instead of the global minimum. Its performance is highly sensitive to the initial relative and suffers from noise and outliers. To overcome such limitations of ICP, some variants of it have been introduced based on the first concept of the ICP algorithm. These variants seek to improve the robustness to noise, speed of convergence, and accuracy of the conventional ICP algorithm by changing and improving the main steps of the ICP algorithm, including selecting points, matching points, weighting pair points, rejecting points, computing the error metric, and minimizing the error metric. In this area, considering selected points instead of all the points by using methods such as downsampling, random sampling, selecting high-intensity points gradient, using distance metrics such as KD trees and Delaunay triangulations instead of Euclidean distance, allocating different weights such as linear fuzzy weight to the corresponding pairs instead of constant weight or rejecting some undesirable pairs, using different error metrics such as point to plane, and also using different optimization methods could improve the accuracy and speed of conventional ICP [69].

Several variations of ICP were applied in different medical applications, including CMF surgery. Recently, in our previous work, one of the variations of the ICP algorithm was proposed to update the normal vector of the plane and find the optimum symmetry plane in reconstruction surgery [69]. The proposed method applied random subsampling and the KD-tree method as a distance metric to find corresponding point-pairs. The KD-tree is a space-partitioning data structure which is used for the organization of points in a k-dimensional space. In this experiment, the registration accuracy was not significantly different from the accuracy of conventional ICP. However, the run-time was reduced by about 99 times. In Fig. 24, the results of the proposed ICP for updating the symmetry plane in ten iterations are shown.

Registration Errors and Error Analysis

As previously noted, a variety of imaging modalities based on the application can be used as preoperative images and fused to patient coordinates, all of which contribute to improved registration accuracy. In addition, there are three types of errors for surgical guidance which affect registration accuracy, including fiducial localization error (FLE), fiducial registration error (FRE), and target registration error (TRE).

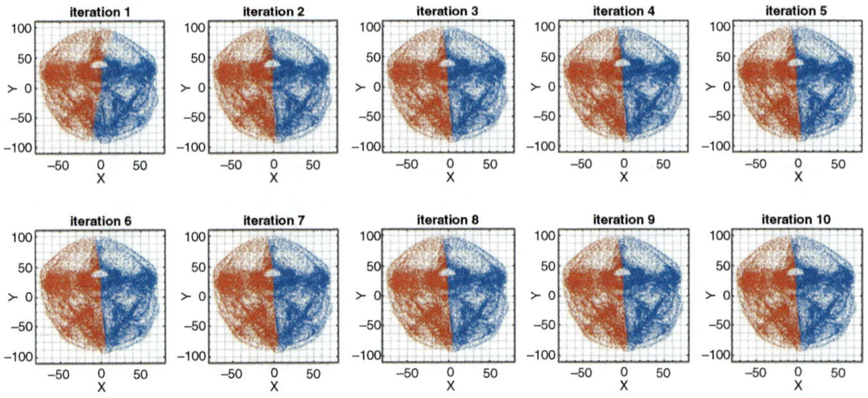

Fig. 24 Visualization of updates in symmetry plane using proposed ICP [69]

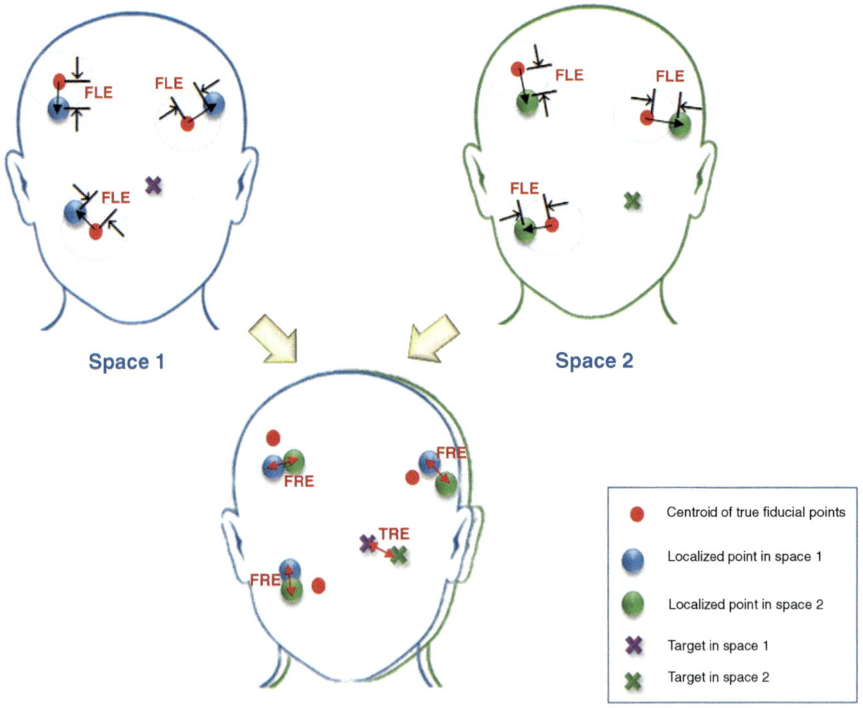

Fig. 25 Illustration of three types of registration errors

The source of all internal errors in the navigation system in both image and reality (operating room) is FLE. As shown in Fig. 25, FLE is the difference vector between actual fiducial positions and incorrectly localized points.

Throughout the registration procedure, matching occurs between the corresponding localized points in the two spaces. After registration, the displacement between corresponding localized points is known as FRE and is calculated with the following equation:

$$\mathrm{FRE} = \sqrt{\frac{1}{N}\sum_{i=1}^{N}\left|p_i^{'} - q_i\right|^2} \tag{1}$$

where N is the number of fiducials and $\left|p_i^{'} - q_i\right|$ represents the distance between a localized fiducial point in space 1 (blue spheres in Fig. 24) and a corresponding localized point in space 2 (green spheres in Fig. 25). According to Eq. (1), it can be inferred that FRE is the root mean square (RMS) of misalignment between registration points. Given that in this equation, non-negative values are added together, it can be inferred that if the FLE is non-zero, there is at least one imperfect aligned registration point [1].

TRE, as the key measure in evaluating the performance of the registration accuracy, and in the following navigation system, is used to assess the accuracy of image-guided interventions that is the distance between corresponding points other than the fiducial points (targets) after registration. The system estimated the TRE using the RMS, which was defined as the distance between the target markers (tm) and the physical targets (pt):

$$\mathrm{TRE} = \left[\left(X_{\mathrm{tm}} - X_{\mathrm{pt}}\right)^2 + \left(Y_{\mathrm{tm}} - Y_{\mathrm{pt}}\right)^2 + \left(Z_{\mathrm{tm}} - Z_{\mathrm{pt}}\right)^2\right]^{1/2} \tag{2}$$

Relation Between Errors

FLE is the source of TRE and FRE. All three errors are statistical in nature, except that FRE is visible and the other two are not visible. Identifying the error relationship can aid in maximizing the navigation system's performance. Although these three errors have no proportionate relationship individually, there are relationships between the RMS value of these errors (which signifies RMS of errors), which can be informative and determined using the equations below.

$$\mathrm{RMS\,TRE}(p) = \frac{1}{\sqrt{N}}\sqrt{1 + \frac{d_1^2}{3f_1^2} + \frac{d_2^2}{3f_2^2} + \frac{d_3^2}{3f_3^2}} \times \mathrm{RMS\,FLE} \tag{3}$$

The proportionality ratio indicates that the RMS TRE in the target p is proportional to the RMS FLE. N denotes the number of fiducials. If the three axes are considered perpendicular to each other in the fiducial configuration's center, d denotes the distance of the target p from each of the axes, and f reflects the orientation with respect to these three axes by computing the RMS distance of N fiducials from one axis and influenced by fiducial shape and size. As a result of this equation,

RMS TRE in the configuration center is the lowest amount because d at the center is zero, and TRE is proportionally related to FLE by ratio $\frac{1}{\sqrt{N}}$.

The RMS FLE can be estimated using the simplified premise that the error probabilities are the same for all fiducials and in all directions in each space, and by considering that RMS FLEs in two spaces are uncorrelated.

$$\text{RMS FLE} = \sqrt{\left(\text{RMS FLE}_{\text{Space1}}\right)^2 + \left(\text{RMS FLE}_{\text{Space2}}\right)^2} \tag{4}$$

The FRE value is returned by current IGS systems as a navigation error. It was discovered that the FRE and TRE values varied significantly in the majority of cases, indicating that FRE is not a reliable measure of error for providing the best registration and precise target localization. When TRE is not possible at the start of the procedure, the surgeon is typically given FRE. On the other hand, this measure does not reflect actual inaccuracy in the target and may perplex the surgeon.

Furthermore, the findings reveal that in a particular fiducial point arrangement, the FRE in targets placed in distinct sinus areas does not change substantially, while the TRE varies significantly depending on the field of surgery.

There are two further statistical relationships that relate RMS FRE to two other errors.

$$\text{RMS FRE} = \sqrt{1-(2/N)} \times \text{RMS FLE} \tag{5}$$

While the shape and configuration of fiducials are very important, they are not apparent in this equation (d,f), and the relationship between RMS FLE and RMS FRE is dictated only by the number of fiducials. The statistical relationship between RMS FLE and RMS TRE can be expressed by combining Eqs. (3) and (5).

$$\text{RMS TRE}(p) = \frac{1}{\sqrt{N-2}}\sqrt{1+\frac{d_1^2}{3f_1^2}+\frac{d_2^2}{3f_2^2}+\frac{d_3^2}{3f_3^2}} \times \text{RMS FRE} \tag{6}$$

RMS TRE at point p is related to RMS FRE by a ratio that relies on the form, configuration, and number of fiducials, according to this equation. This may be deduced from the formula, which asserts that moving some of the fiducials around the target will change the RMS TRE value in a particular region for any fiducial distribution patterns.

3 Registration Accuracy Improvement

There are different approaches which improve the accuracy of image registration, such as changing the number of landmarks, different landmark configurations, using different patterns, touchless registration, and advanced registration algorithms. In the following, these approaches will be discussed.

Landmark Configuration

One of the main approaches which is used for this purpose is applying different numbers and configurations of landmarks. Reliable tracking of surgical tools for accurate navigation is achieved by precise target localization using fiducial landmarks, which can be performed invasively or noninvasively in several head and neck surgeries. As discussed before, anatomical landmarks are more common due to their ease of implementation, noninvasiveness, and naturalness. The accuracy of the TRE significantly depends on the number of fiducials, their distribution, and exact localization. To reduce TRE, it is recommended to use more fiducials and a nonlinear layout. Therefore, in our previous works, different numbers and configurations of landmarks were applied in different fields of surgery, such as bronchoscopy [70], spine surgery [71], dental surgery [72], and also CMF [65], and finally, the optimal arrangements were proposed for each. In Table 5, the effect of different configurations using four landmarks in image-guided spine surgery was investigated, and TREs by considering equal weights for landmarks were measured. Markers were inserted in the pedicle of the vertebra as the objective in this study was to estimate registration accuracy during pedicle screw insertion surgery using navigation. The measured TRE in the third column is the best TRE, but the second configuration due to covering the whole surface to be registered was considered as the optimum configuration of landmarks during the surgery.

In another study, to investigate the best configurations of anatomical landmarks for image-guided dental implant surgery, a dental phantom consisting of implanted targets was used. As shown in Fig. 26, the target points were located in six operation sites, which nearly covered selected implant surgery targets.

The best configuration of landmarks in image-guided dental surgery to obtain minimum TRE in each target region is illustrated in Table 6. TRE is reported in the table as the mean squared distance between a target point in image space and the probe point approaching the homologous target point in physical space.

The general recommendation for TRE reduction is to arrange the fiducials sparsely around the surgical target, so that the center of gravity is closer to the surgical target. However, in practice, this essential suggestion necessitates more specific guidance. Also, adding more anatomical landmarks or avoiding collinear configuration is less significant than optimizing landmark configuration to minimize TRE value.

Table 5 Effect of different configurations using four landmarks in image-guided spine surgery [71]

Landmark configuration	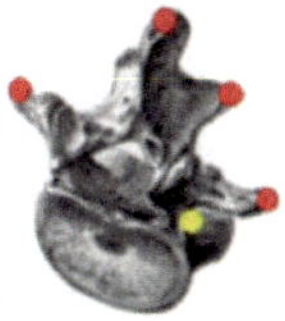	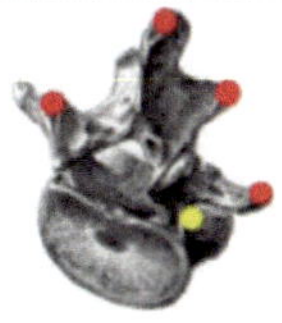	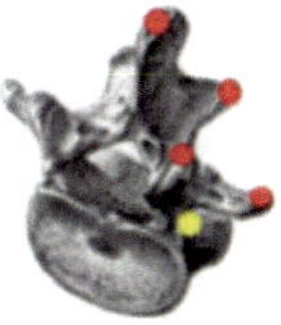	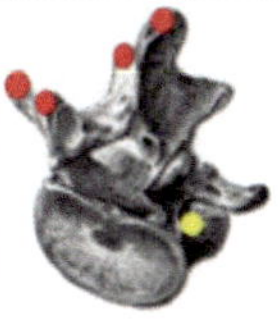
Measured TRE (mm)	1.0688	1.0682	0.9532	1.5116

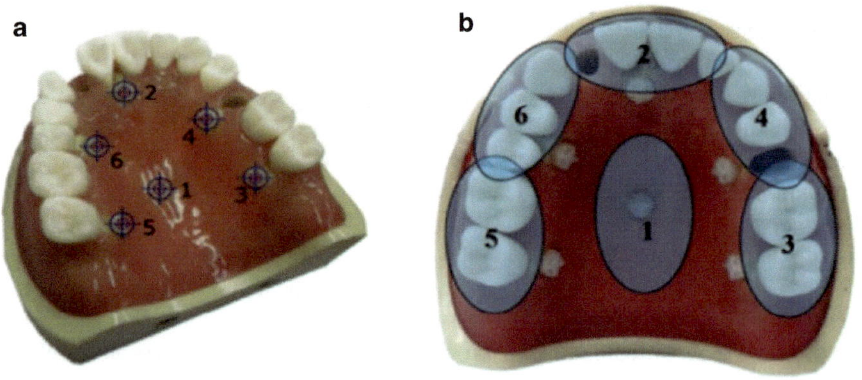

Fig. 26 (**a**) Six targets with their numbers on phantom and (**b**) the target regions covered by implanted markers in image-guided dental surgery [72]

Table 6 The best configuration of landmarks to reach minimum TRE in each dental target

Target region	T1	T2	T3	T4	T5	T6
Best configuration	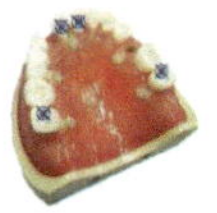	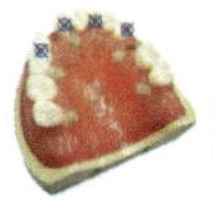	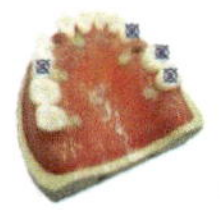	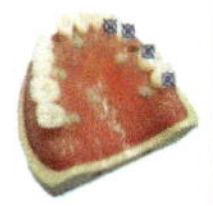	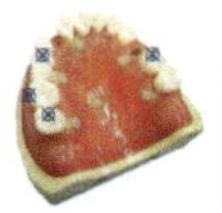	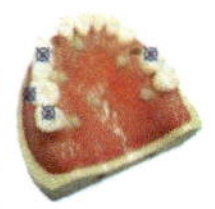
TRE (mm)	0.104	0.130	0.341	0.532	0.319	0.410

For the best selection of fiducials, the configurations are organized around the following crucial details:

1. Avoiding nearly linear fiducial placement.
2. Keeping fiducials properly far apart.
3. Picking more points surrounding the target area.
4. Placing fiducials on the most inflexible anatomical points, such as the nasal bridge, canthi of the eyes, and tragi of the ears.

For accurate navigation in the four areas of sinus surgery, in [65], the FRE and TRE values were measured in a different configuration of landmarks over the frontal, ethmoid, sphenoid, and maxillary regions, and optimum fiducial configuration patterns were proposed.

The nasal bridge landmark is easy to detect and its central location on the face gives a good area to adjust the middle of the fiducials. The following seven-point patterns represent the mean TRE values in four indicated areas. Because the sphenoid targets are on both sides of the head, TRE might be lowered by centering the fiducials in the middle and adding two points on both sides of the nose (see Fig. 27).

A four-point pattern is shown in Fig. 28. The fiducials in this pattern are centered on the frontal region, and there seems no need to add any further points to this pattern. Thus, this pattern was investigated over the frontal region.

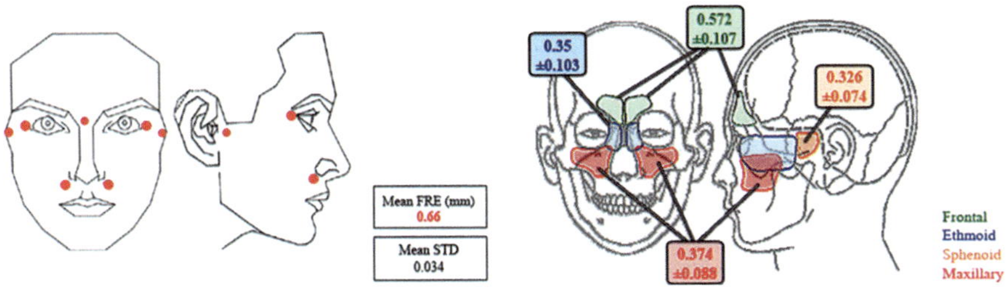

Fig. 27 The FRE and TRE values were measured over the frontal, ethmoid, sphenoid, and maxillary regions of the sinus area in a seven-point pattern [65]

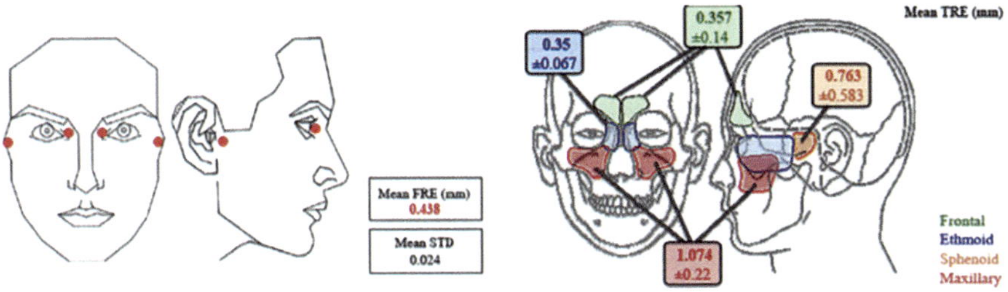

Fig. 28 The FRE and TRE values were measured over the frontal, ethmoid, sphenoid, and maxillary regions of sinus area in a four-point pattern [65]

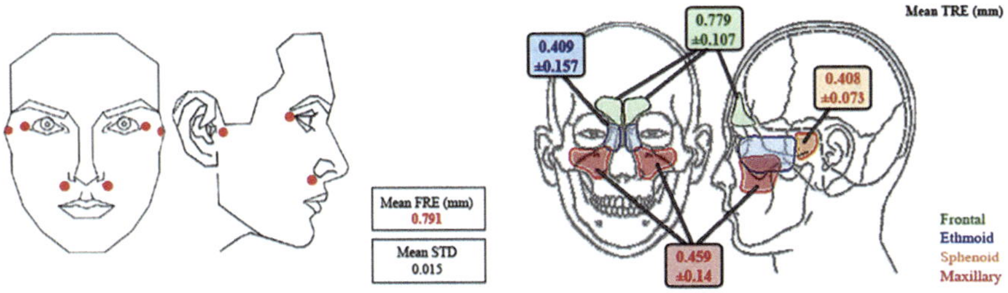

Fig. 29 The FRE and TRE values were measured over the frontal, ethmoid, sphenoid, and maxillary regions of sinus area in a six-point pattern [65]

In order to create a balance on the surface being registered, the canthi of the eyes are frequently used. For example, Fig. 29 represents a six-point pattern with two fiducials on the canthi of the eyes. This pattern is one of the best choices in the ethmoid, maxillary, and sphenoid regions by reducing the TRE values.

The eight-point pattern is made by inserting two landmarks into the preview pattern, spreading the fiducials more over the frontal region. The impact of increasing the number of fiducials on decreasing the TRE value may be analyzed using an eight-point pattern (Fig. 30).

All of these studies indicate the need to optimize the numbers and arrangement of the landmarks corresponding to the surgical field. Also, results proved that the landmark configuration is more effective at reducing TRE value than adding anatomical landmarks or avoiding collinear configuration.

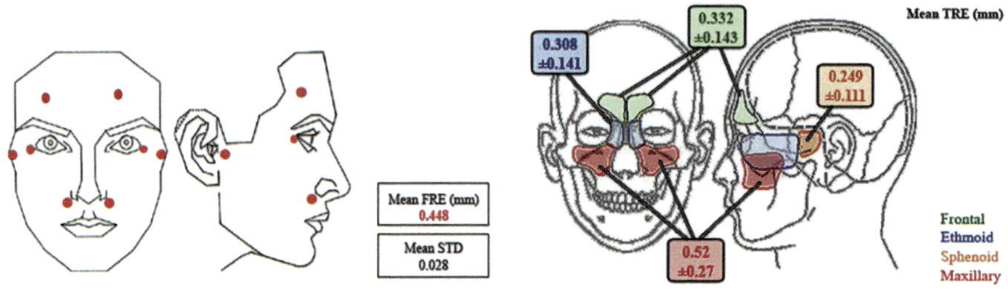

Fig. 30 The FRE and TRE values were measured over the frontal, ethmoid, sphenoid, and maxillary regions of the sinus area in an eight-point pattern [65]

Accurate Landmark Selection

Another one of the main approaches which is used to increase registration accuracy is accurate marker selection during the navigation process. In navigation systems, the anatomy and spatial orientation of the patient must be registered with the preoperative images. Landmarks are used to precisely define the patient's three-dimensional location in space during the registration procedure. This is done in two ways: touch-based and touchless approaches.

Touch-Based Methods

In the touch-based approaches, we focused on accurate selection and localization of the fiducial markers which are used during the registration process through tool tip contact with critical points. Selecting anatomic and bony landmarks such as the tragus, teeth, or eye corners by using a navigation tool tip is a common way to achieve accurate registration. Alternatively, moving a navigation tool tip over the skin's surface results in a large number of fiducials being accumulated for patient registration. Furthermore, attachment of fiducial markers such as screws to the skin before preoperative imaging is a strategy for accurate registration. Regardless of simple procedures, all these approaches are time-consuming and prone to human error and FLE errors.

In the CMF field, splints which contain fiducial markers are used for registration. To make this clear, consider orthognathic surgery, which is done by using a surgical navigation system to correct facial asymmetry. The accuracy of surgical navigation is dependent on registration accuracy, which is highly affected by the repositioning process. Using a common splint during these surgeries and selecting markers on it is prone to errors. In our recent work, a novel-designed splint integrated with a star-shaped navigation frame and fiducial markers and jointly printed for orthognathic bimaxillary surgery was proposed. Fiducial markers are designed in such a way that the navigation tool tip fits properly on them to minimize fiducial localization errors. Also, using fewer fiducial markers and proper spatial distribution lead to speeding

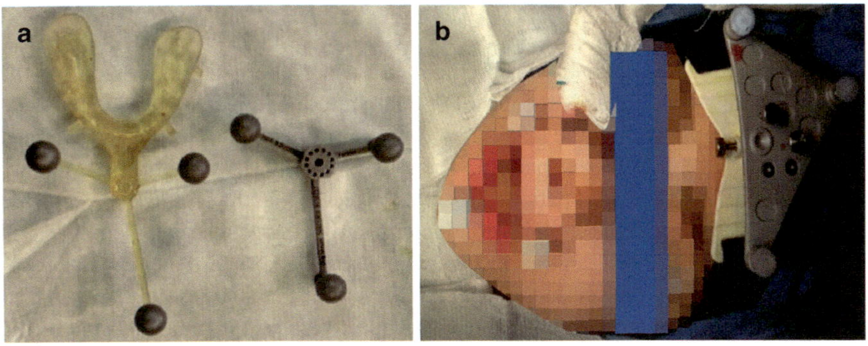

Fig. 31 (**a**) Novel designed splint, (**b**) Intraoperative view which is showing the positioning of novel designed splint

up the registration procedure and reducing registration errors, respectively. These novel designed splints are applicable mainly to cases of bimaxillary orthognathic surgery. In 2021, a 21-year-old woman with malocclusion class II and vertically maxillary excess was scheduled for bimaxillary surgery using computer-assisted planning and surgical navigation (Fig. 31). To find the accurate location of the maxilla, the splint should be tracked using the navigation system. Therefore, reflective spherical markers are attached to the star-shaped navigation frame. In the point-to-point registration procedure, points were extracted by placing the navigation tool on the fiducial markers printed on the splint and then were registered in the navigation system. The total time of the registration procedure considering splint setting is less than 20 s, approximately. As the novel-designed splint is printed seamlessly, it is very lightweight and stable. Therefore, there is no additional error imposed by the splint on the navigation system. The fiducial registration error was less than 0.5 mm in point-to-point registration.

Touchless Methods

The registration methods mentioned in the previous part require the presence of fiducial markers in the preoperative images. Because of the tool pressure on body skin in the conventional registration methods, the likelihood of patient registration errors is increased. Touchless registration is an alternative to touch-based or marker-based registration, which is time-consuming and prone to human error, among other drawbacks [73]. These methods are meant to improve registration accuracy by reducing the FLE errors as mentioned before. There are different approaches to considering touchless registration methods which improve the accuracy of image registration, such as using optical patterns, laser pointer scanners, and 3D scanners. In the following, we first discuss optical pattern registration, and then laser pointer and 3D scanner approaches will be discussed.

Optical Patterns

Among the touchless registration methods, a proper alternative approach for the acquisition of point clouds is the use of optical patterns projected onto the patient's body. In these approaches, the landmark points on surfaces are selected and sampled by projecting a checkerboard pattern. Then, by using a CCD camera, the conjunction points of the checkered pattern, so-called projected landmarks, will be detected [74]. Finally, surface registration is conducted via the 3D reconstructed points cloud created by the Projected Landmarks by scaling the checkerboard elements or scanning a pattern across the surface to meet the appropriate spatial resolution; the number of selected points could be defined and controlled in this manner. Due to the pattern projection on the desired region, fewer points are needed and the effects of unwanted and overlapping points can be eliminated. In our previous work [74], different patterns considering anatomical areas such as the nose, lips, and the forehead for ENT surgery were evaluated (see Fig. 32). The patterns are projected on the phantom using a light source, such as a projector, which is demonstrated in Fig. 33.

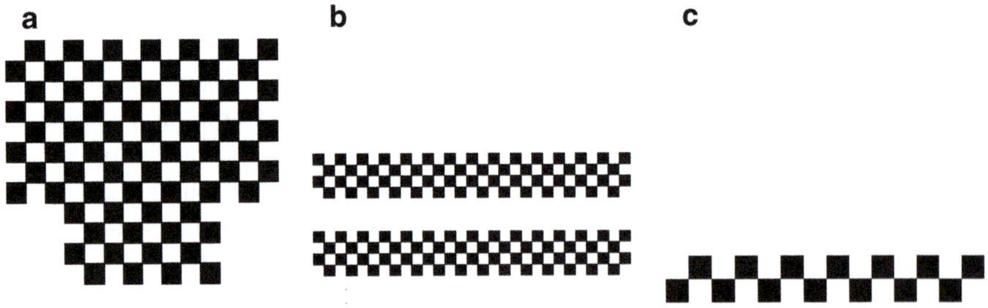

Fig. 32 Different patterns for capturing the curvatures of the face. Pattern (**a**) is designed to capture the curvatures of the nose and lips, (**b**) is designed to capture the curvatures of the forehead and nose, (**c**) is designed to capture of the points on both the sides of the nose [74]

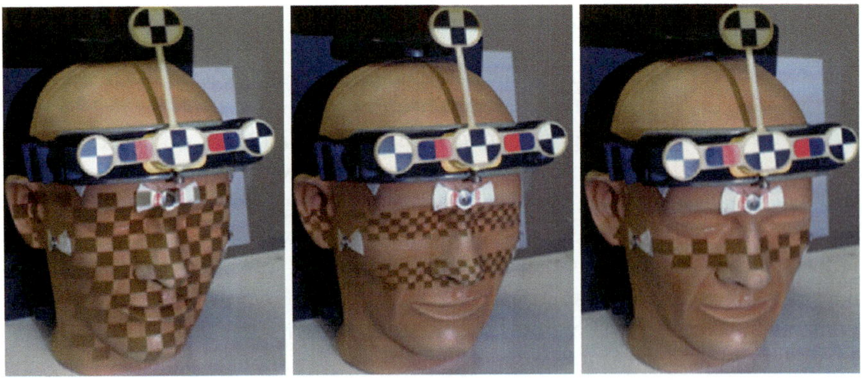

Fig. 33 Examples of projecting different patterns on different regions of interest [74]

Laser Pointer and 3D Scanner

The touchless registration methods based on laser and 3D scanners are fast and reliable. In this procedure, face skin surface scanning is done by a laser pointer or 3D scanner. The provided point clouds from the laser pointer or 3D scanner are then registered by preoperative captured images. Using point clouds collected from a laser pointer or 3D scanner can provide the following advantages:

1. Improving the registration accuracy and the speed of registration setup by scanning patient surfaces with a pointer or scanner to capture a large number of surface points in a short period of time.
2. Improving the navigation accuracy by reducing the FLE errors caused by not touching the patient's skin.
3. Lesser needs to have an expert technician in the operating room to handle the patient registration process as a key part of the image-guided navigation system.
4. Due to contact with the patient's skin surface, the tools used intraoperatively in the registration process are not sterile and are not acceptable for use in the next procedure. The touchless registration method eliminates the requirement for using two different sets of registration and navigation instruments, as well as making the patient more comfortable with less infection risk.

Therefore, the main purpose of using these tools is to achieve high-precision point clouds, more patient comfort, increasing navigation accuracy, speed of data collection, reduced infection risk, reproducibility of the process during surgery, and, as a result, ease of use of the system in OR by medical staff. Z-touch® (BrainLab) and FAZER (Medtronic Xomed) have been used in studies for touch-less registration (laser pointer). Studies have showed that surface registration with laser scanning is an accurate, robust, effective, and efficient way of patient registration for navigation [75].

Additionally, the integration of 3D scanners into image-guided platforms will be a promising future development [76]. In a recent study, a portable 3D scanner was used to acquire a marker less patient-to-image registration [77] and proved as a promising surface-acquisition device. However, laser scanners as a proper alternative to other methods save registration time. Laser scanners are popular among touchless scanning methods due to their low cost. Laser scanners are popular among touchless scanning methods due to their low cost (Fig. 34).

Registration Algorithm Improvement

One of the main approaches to improving registration accuracy is the development of novel registration algorithms. Since the navigation system applies a point-based registration method, we focused on these registration techniques, briefly. As we discussed, ICP is a distance-based method commonly used in navigation systems. After the introduction of ICP and its variants, some probabilistic-based methods,

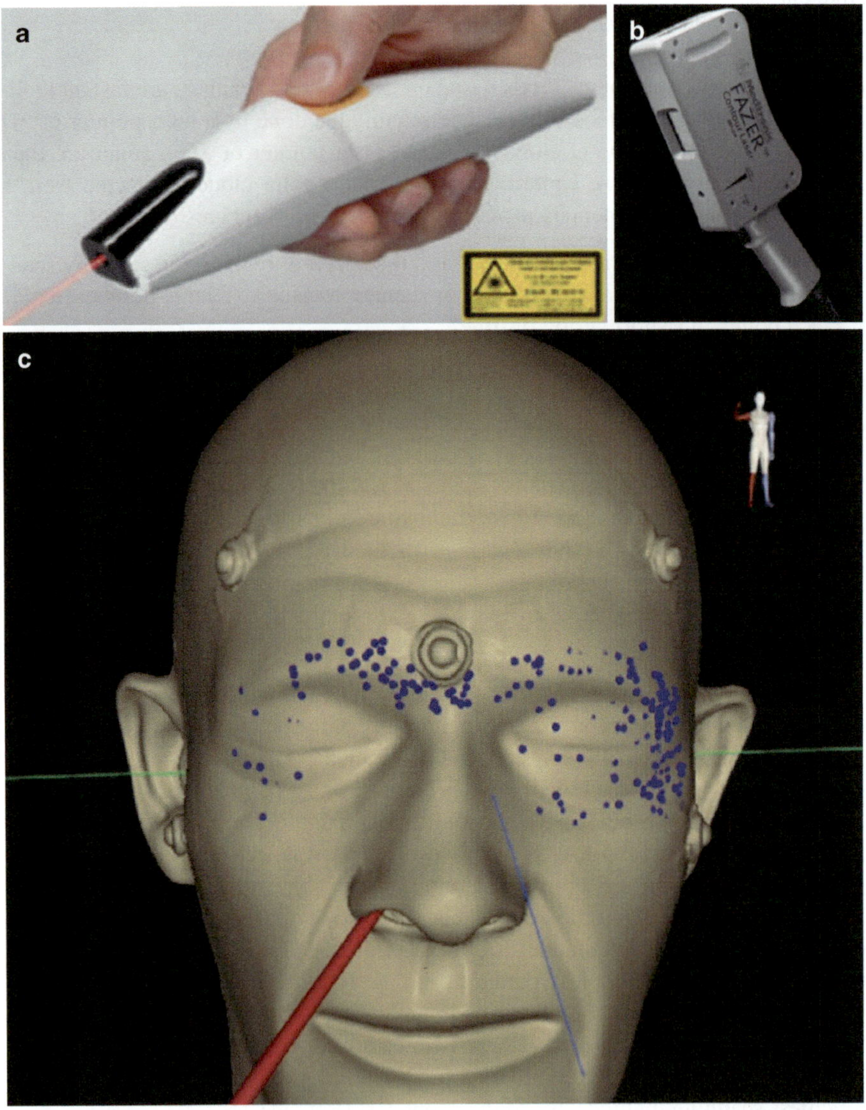

Fig. 34 The pointer laser devices used in patient touchless registration. (**a**) Z-touch (Brainlab, Germany), (**b**) FAZER (Medtronic Xomed), (**c**) Point clouds acquired by surface scanning by laser pointer on phantom (provided by Parsiss Co.). Surface scanning with a laser pointer on a phantom obtained point clouds

such as the robust point matching method (RPM) [78], Gaussian mixture model (GMM) [79], and coherent point drift method (CPD) [80] were proposed to overcome the limitations of distance-based methods and increase the registration accuracy. The CPD, as one of the most successful point-based registration algorithms, is considered as a probability density estimation problem, where one-point set represents the GMM centroids and the other one the data points. Therefore, the maximum of GMM posterior probability is obtained when the two-point sets are matched. Many studies investigated different variations of CPD, especially in non-rigid problems, to improve its performance in different fields, such as image-guided surgery [81, 82]. Furthermore, recently, some hybrid registration methods which use intensity and features of images simultaneously have been introduced to increase registration accuracy.

4 Limitations and Some Cures for Surgical Navigation Systems

Soft Tissue Deformation and Intraoperative Imaging

Soft tissue deformation is the main source of error that happens during surgery, affects the surgical navigation systems accuracy, and invalidates preoperative images in different fields of surgery, such as neurosurgery, abdomen surgery, and CMF. This phenomenon still remains as the current challenging problem in performing a highly accurate image-guided navigation surgery.

Neurosurgery is one of the main areas of surgery that is faced with soft tissue deformation. Maximal safe resection of brain tumors in eloquent regions is optimally performed under IGS systems. The accuracy of the image-guided neurosurgery system is drastically affected by intraoperative tissue deformation of the brain, called brain shift. Brain shift is a dynamic, complex, and spatiotemporal phenomenon which happens after performing a craniotomy and invalidates the preoperative image of patients. The brain shift, which is known as the brain deformation, is a combination of a wide variety of biological, physical, and surgical causes and occurs in both cortical and deep brain structures. Brain shift calculation and compensation methods are based on updating the preoperative images with regard to the intraoperative tissue deformation. These methods fall into three main categories: biomechanical modeling, intraoperative imaging approaches, and hybrid methods, which combine biomechanical models with intraoperative imaging [81]. Biomechanical model-based as highly accurate approaches are time-consuming methods. The main challenge of model-based methods is that the tissue deformations that occur during intraoperative neuro-surgical procedures are hard to real-time accurately model and thus are often not considered [83]. Therefore, most recent studies have focused on using intraoperative imaging, including intraoperative computed tomography (CT), MRI, fluorescence-guided surgery, and ultrasound (US) imaging during neurosurgery [84].

CT images, as one of the primary modalities which are used intraoperatively, suffer from lower soft tissue contrast compared to MRI; therefore, intraoperative CT images are less functional for brain surgery. Although new approaches for reducing the exposure to the patient and OR staff have been proposed, the radiation dose to the patient is one of the most important limitations of using CT scans in OR. Besides, the physical space occupied by the CT scanner in the OR is another problem. The intraoperative MRI with the best soft tissue contrast compared to the other imaging modalities is not real-time imaging. However, intraoperative MRI is considered as the gold standard for intraoperative imaging, but it requires a dedicated intraoperative MRI suite and an equipped operating room with MR-compatible instruments [85]. Ultrasound, the alternative imaging system, has a long history of intraoperative use in different surgeries, such as prostate, breast, and liver surgery. Although intraoperative US imaging has been slow to enter the field of neurosurgery, it remains an effective solution for many challenging problems in this field. In recent years, intraoperative US has been used for many procedures such as biopsy, tumor localization, and determining the tumor or the tissue margin in many patients who undergo neurosurgery due to its advantages, such as being non-ionized, inexpensive, real-time, portable, and operating room equipment compatibility. One of the most important applications of intraoperative US imaging is calculating and compensating for brain shift, which invalidates preoperative image coordination [86]. Intraoperative fluorescence imaging as optical imaging enables real-time intraoperative delineation of glioma tissue. The 5-aminolevulinic acid as an accepted composite for this imaging is a non-fluorescent agent which is converted to fluorescent within the tumor cells. The main advantage of this modality is its high contrast to differentiate malignant and normal brain tissue. This method has shortcomings, such as skin photosensitivity, dependent on imaging depth, and time because fluorescence signals can be obscured by upper tissues and the passing of time [87].

Totally, the integration of navigation systems and intraoperative imaging is a well-established technique to acquire real-time images, compensate for tissue deformation, and guide surgical procedures accurately. Despite numerous imaging modalities, there is still a requirement for the development of navigation systems by using new imaging systems to overcome the limitations of conventional imaging. Photoacoustic imaging (PAI) has been proven to have tremendous potential in medical imaging for preclinical and clinical applications, such as functional brain mapping, cancer diagnosis, and staging [88], tissue vasculature [89, 90], oral health [91, 92], and image-guided surgeries [93, 94]. In the PAI processes, the tissue illuminated by the nanosecond time scale pulsed light, then absorbed optical energy led to increase in local temperature and consequently expand the tissue which generates wideband ultrasound waves. Affected by this phenomenon, the endogenous chromophores such as hemoglobin provide intense photoacoustic signals due to high optical absorption coefficients, and therefore, crucial structural information such as blood vessels and tumor angiogenesis is demonstrated by using PAI [95, 96]. The PAI combines optical and ultrasound imaging modalities based on the photoacoustic effect phenomenon to achieve the contrast of optical imaging as well as the spatial resolution of ultrasound imaging [97, 98]. Since PAI uses US signals generated by the absorbers inside the tissue, it enables imaging of relatively deep absorbers in the tissue compared to pure optical imaging techniques (see Fig. 35). Considering all these advantages, using intraoperative PAI was proposed recently in 2020, for brain shift correction [99, 100]. Also, due to the advantages and high

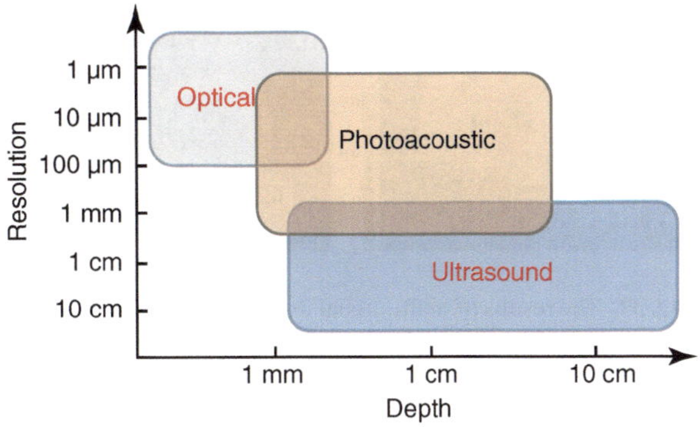

Fig. 35 Comparison of the resolution and depth among different imaging modalities: ultrasound, optical, and photoacoustic imaging [90]

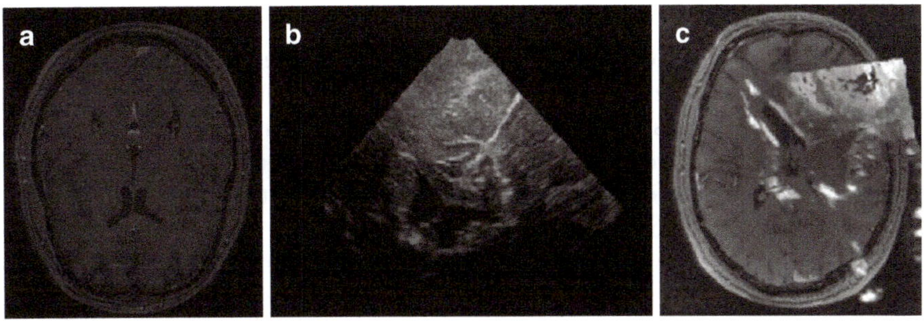

Fig. 36 The results of multi-modal image registration of brain to calculate brain shift. (**a**) Preoperative MRI, (**b**) Intraoperative ultrasound, and (**c**) Registration of deformed US and MRI of brain [86]

efficiency of PAI, many studies are trying to improve the quality of these images more, via improving signal de-noising [101] or image reconstruction approaches [99, 102].

As we discussed, despite all the advantages and disadvantages of all intraoperative imaging, interventional imaging systems are becoming an integral part of modern surgery to update patients' coordinates during surgery using registration of intraoperative images with preoperative images. However, finding a single satisfactory solution for registration of intraoperative images with preoperative images is a challenging task due to the complex and unpredictable nature of the deformation during surgery. Many investigations have tried to overcome the limitations of image registration algorithms, especially in multi-modal registration cases, in processes of soft tissue compensation. There are many studies trying to improve registration accuracy for multi-modal image registration, including feature-based methods, intensity-based methods, and hybrid methods simultaneously using features and intensity pixels (102). In the following, two examples of ultrasound-MR image registration (Fig. 36) and photoacoustic-MR image registration (Fig. 37) have been shown.

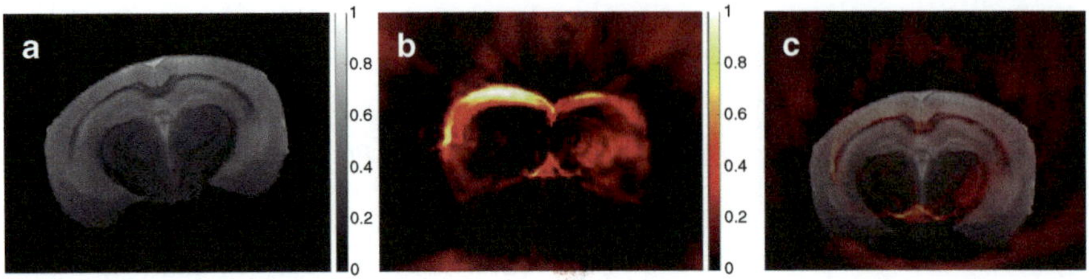

Fig. 37 The results of multi-modal image registration of mouse brain data. (**a**) MRI, (**b**) PA image after deformation, and (**c**) Registration of deformed PA and MRI of mouse data [100]

Intraoperative Validation of Surgical Navigation Using Intraoperative Imaging

Surgical navigation systems are now increasingly being used for the guidance of numerous surgeries. Despite the clinical advantages of surgical navigation, it has drawbacks since it relies on preoperative imaging data. Therefore, some procedures, such as head and neck resection and reconstruction surgeries due to morphological changes owing to surgical excision, anatomical deformation, and tumor growth need to be evaluated during the surgery. This intraoperative evaluation is usually done using intraoperative imaging. For example, to quantify the accuracy of osteotomy navigation for mandible and maxilla resection, CBCT-guided surgery was proposed [103] (Fig. 38). In this important study, CBCT-guided osteotomy navigation was performed pre-clinically on five cadaver heads with a mean FRE of about 0.5 mm, and also on five patients with mean of FRE of about 0.7 mm. Totally, CBCT-guided surgical navigation achieved a mean cutting accuracy of less than 2 mm.

5 Future Prospects

The IGS systems cover a broad range of minimally invasive surgeries (MIS) which lead to surgical trauma reduction such as wound infections, pain and hernias, shorter hospitalizations, and quick return to routine life [104]. Technological advances in some existing areas, like virtual and augmented reality, robotics, and artificial intelligence (AI), hold promises in IGS. This information improves surgical planning and guides the surgeon during the surgical procedures.

Technological innovations in augmented reality (AR), virtual reality (VR), and mixed reality (MR) have led to emerging navigational solutions in IGS [105]. AR is a technology which overlays virtual data onto the real world and allows the surgeon to precisely and efficiently interact with the physical environment while navigational information is provided on the operative field. In contrast, VR provides an immersive virtual computer-generated environment where users through a

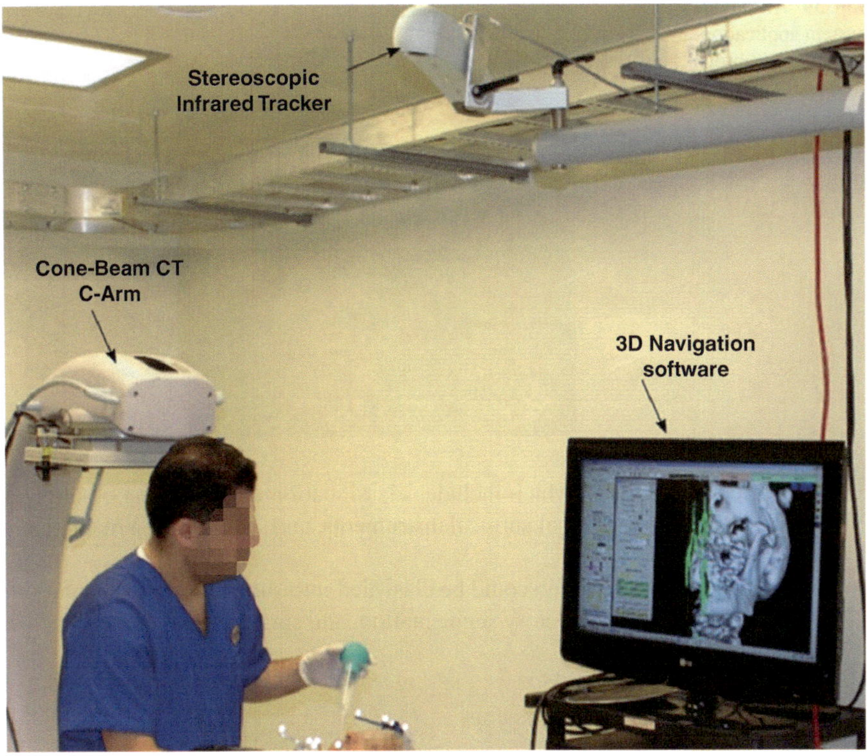

Fig. 38 CBCT-guided osteotomy navigation [103]

head-mounted display (HMD), haptic feedback devices, and haptic gloves in real-time interact with the virtual environment [106]. MR is a continuum between real and virtual worlds in which virtual and physical data interact with each other in this shared environment [107]. Medical image processing approaches provide 3D models of patients derived from preoperative CT or MRI images. Applying AR during surgical operations superimposes the 3D models onto the patient's physical space and allows the surgeon to have interactive and dynamic visualization. Real-time surgical tool navigation techniques help them to track surgical tools in enhanced reality views. An example of AR navigation system application in craniofacial fibrous dysplasia surgery is shown in Fig. 39. Through the HMD, the surgeon can see the craniofacial skull and lesion images, the surgical field, and the location of surgical tools in real time [108].

In recent years, artificial intelligence, particularly deep learning approaches, has attracted great attention for various applications in medical areas, such as image segmentation [109], image reconstruction [99], and image de-noising [110]. One of the most important applications of deep learning is in computer-assisted diagnostic systems, including navigation and IGS systems to perform MIS, which has opened the following approaches [111]:

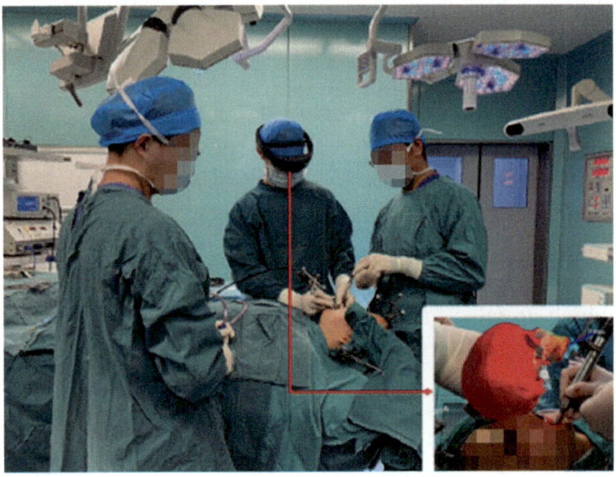

Fig. 39 AR navigation system application in craniofacial fibrous dysplasia surgery [108]

- Surgical image analysis, which includes classification and detection of surgical instruments, segmentation of surgical instruments, and segmentation of anatomical structures.
- Surgical task analysis, which could be classified into surgical phase recognition, gesture segmentation, trajectory segmentation, and surgery time prediction.
- Surgical skill assessment.
- Automation of surgical tasks.
- Intelligent surgical training systems.

Enormous work has been done in the above-mentioned areas, and the results are so promising. However, it seems that in the next 10 years, artificial intelligence methods will create a revolution in image-guided navigation systems. Based on our understanding, there are two reasons for this claim. The first one is the high volume of medical data. However, many texts state that the volume of medical data is smaller than that in other fields, which could be a challenge for network training. But in fact, there is a large amount of medical data in various fields that has remained practically useless. The problem of network training with medical data can also be solved by developing a network architecture. On the other hand, processes such as image segmentation, which are performed manually by the physician in most medical processes, are very time-consuming. For example, the process of facial bone segmentation to design a surgical plan wastes about one day. While, deep learning approaches can enable network training based on physician knowledge as a gold standard in combination with conventional methods. In this way, physician knowledge is learned over times by networks.

Also, robotic surgery technology aims at helping surgeons to deliver more accuracy and precision during complicated surgeries [112]. Integrating with surgical planning and navigation systems, robotic arms are localized and controlled in a 3D space. Additionally, AI expert systems as smart surgery assistants in the near future will be used in IGS to store and have meaningful insight into large amounts of medical information while they are able to interact with surgeons [113].

References

1. Citardi MJ. In: Labadie R, Fitzpatrick JM, editors. Image-guided surgery: fundamentals and clinical applications in otolaryngology. San Diego, CA: Plural Publishing; 2016, 215 pp.
2. Wang JC, Nagy L, Demke JC. Image-guided surgery and craniofacial applications: mastering the unseen. Maxillofac Plast Reconst Surg. 2015;37(1):1–5.
3. Bessen SY, Wu X, Sramek MT, Shi Y, Pastel D, Halter R, et al. Image-guided surgery in otolaryngology: a review of current applications and future directions in head and neck surgery. Head Neck. 2021;43(8):2534–53.
4. Schmale IL, Vandelaar LJ, Luong AU, Citardi MJ, Yao WC. Image-guided surgery and intraoperative imaging in rhinology: clinical update and current state of the art. Ear Nose Throat J. 2021;100(10):NP475–86.
5. García-Mato D, Ochandiano S, García-Sevilla M, Navarro-Cuéllar C, Darriba-Allés JV, García-Leal R, et al. Craniosynostosis surgery: workflow based on virtual surgical planning, intraoperative navigation and 3D printed patient-specific guides and templates. Sci Rep. 2019;9(1):1–10.
6. Kaduk W, Podmelle F, Louis PJ. Surgical navigation in reconstruction. Oral Maxillofac Surg Clin North Am. 2013;25(2):313–33.
7. Luz M, Strauss G, Manzey D. Impact of image-guided surgery on surgeons' performance: a literature review. Int J Hum Factors Ergon. 2016;4(3–4):229–63.
8. Silva D, Belsuzarri T, Barnett GH. Image-guided surgery for meningioma. In: Handbook of clinical neurology, vol. 170. Elsevier; 2020. p. 201–7.
9. Eggers G, Mühling J, Hofele C. Clinical use of navigation based on cone-beam computer tomography in maxillofacial surgery. Br J Oral Maxillofac Surg. 2009;47(6):450–4.
10. Anne Woloshyn T. Soaking up the rays: Light therapy and visual culture in Britain, c. 1890–1940. Manchester: Manchester University Press; 2017.
11. Kyriakides Y. Accuracy assessment of a novel optical image guided system for trans-nasal sinus and skull base surgeries. Int Bull Otorhinolaryngol. 2020;16(2):41–5.
12. Rahman M, Murad GJ, Mocco J. Early history of the stereotactic apparatus in neurosurgery. Neurosurg Focus. 2009;27(3):E12.
13. Jensen RL, Stone JL, Hayne RA. Introduction of the human Horsley-Clarke stereotactic frame. Neurosurgery. 1996;38(3):563–7.
14. Henderson JM, Holloway KL, Gaede SE, Rosenow JM. The application accuracy of a skull-mounted trajectory guide system for image-guided functional neurosurgery. Comput Aided Surg. 2004;9(4):155–60.
15. Vogele M, Freysinger W, Bale R, Gunkel A, Thumfart W. Einsatz der ISG Viewing Wand am Felsenbein Eine Modellstudie. HNO. 1997;45(2):74–80.
16. Haßfeld S, Mühling J, Zöller J. Intraoperative navigation in oral and maxillofacial surgery. Int J Oral Maxillofac Surg. 1995;24(1):111–9.
17. Bell RB. Computer planning and intraoperative navigation in cranio-maxillofacial surgery. Oral Maxillofac Surg Clin. 2010;22(1):135–56.
18. Hammer B, Kunz C, Schramm A, Prein J. Repair of complex orbital fractures: technical problems, state-of-the-art solutions and future perspectives. Ann Acad Med Singap. 1999;28(5):687–91.
19. Marmulla R, Niederdellmann H. Computer-assisted bone segment navigation. J Cranio-Maxillofac Surg. 1998;26(6):347–59.
20. Tatli U, Evlice B. Cone-beam computed tomography for oral and maxillofacial imaging. In: Computed tomography: advanced applications. Rijeka: InTech; 2017. p. 139.
21. Zhao M, Wang L, Chen J, Nie D, Cong Y, Ahmad S, et al., editors. Craniomaxillofacial bony structures segmentation from MRI with deep-supervision adversarial learning. International conference on medical image computing and computer-assisted intervention. Springer;2018.
22. Scarfe WC, Li Z, Aboelmaaty W, Scott S, Farman A. Maxillofacial cone beam computed tomography: essence, elements and steps to interpretation. Aust Dent J. 2012;57:46–60.

23. Lee Y-H, Lee KM, Auh Q. MRI-based assessment of masticatory muscle changes in TMD patients after whiplash injury. J Clin Med. 2021;10(7):1404.
24. Yilmaz HH, Yildirim D, Ugan Y, Tunc SE, Yesildag A, Orhan H, et al. Clinical and magnetic resonance imaging findings of the temporomandibular joint and masticatory muscles in patients with rheumatoid arthritis. Rheumatol Int. 2012;32(5):1171–8.
25. Karumuri SK, Rastogi T, Beeraka K, Penumatcha MR, Olepu SR. Ultrasound: a revenant therapeutic modality in dentistry. J Clin Diagn Res. 2016;10(7):ZE08.
26. Slak B, Daabous A, Bednarz W, Strumban E, Maev RG. Assessment of gingival thickness using an ultrasonic dental system prototype: a comparison to traditional methods. Ann Anat. 2015;199:98–103.
27. Gsaxner C, Wallner J, Chen X, Zemann W, Egger J. Facial model collection for medical augmented reality in oncologic cranio-maxillofacial surgery. Sci Data. 2019;6(1):1–7.
28. Nardi C, Molteni R, Lorini C, Taliani GG, Matteuzzi B, Mazzoni E, et al. Motion artefacts in cone beam CT: an in vitro study about the effects on the images. Br J Radiol. 2016;89(1058):20150687.
29. Nardi C, Borri C, Regini F, Calistri L, Castellani A, Lorini C, et al. Metal and motion artifacts by cone beam computed tomography (CBCT) in dental and maxillofacial study. Radiol Med. 2015;120(7):618–26.
30. Schulze R, Heil U, Groβ D, Bruellmann D, Dranischnikow E, Schwanecke U, et al. Artefacts in CBCT: a review. Dentomaxillofac Radiol. 2011;40(5):265–73.
31. Bhoosreddy AR, Sakhavalkar PU. Image deteriorating factors in cone beam computed tomography, their classification, and measures to reduce them: a pictorial essay. J Indian Acad Oral Med Radiol. 2014;26(3):293.
32. Makins SR. Artifacts interfering with interpretation of cone beam computed tomography images. Dent Clin N Am. 2014;58(3):485–95.
33. Barrett JF, Keat N. Artifacts in CT: recognition and avoidance. Radiographics. 2004;24(6):1679–91.
34. Fox A, Basrani B, Kishen A, Lam EW. A novel method for characterizing beam hardening artifacts in cone-beam computed tomographic images. J Endod. 2018;44(5):869–74.
35. Nagarajappa AK, Dwivedi N, Tiwari R. Artifacts: the downturn of CBCT image. J Int Soc Prev Community Dent. 2015;5(6):440.
36. Hong J, Hashizume M. An effective point-based registration tool for surgical navigation. Surg Endosc. 2010;24(4):944–8.
37. Zhou Z, Wu B, Duan J, Zhang X, Zhang N, Liang Z. Optical surgical instrument tracking system based on the principle of stereo vision. J Biomed Opt. 2017;22(6):065005.
38. Sorriento A, Porfido MB, Mazzoleni S, Calvosa G, Tenucci M, Ciuti G, et al. Optical and electromagnetic tracking systems for biomedical applications: a critical review on potentialities and limitations. IEEE Rev Biomed Eng. 2019;13:212–32.
39. Kügler D, Krumb H, Bredemann J, Stenin I, Kristin J, Klenzner T, et al. High-precision evaluation of electromagnetic tracking. Int J Comput Assist Radiol Surg. 2019;14(7):1127–35.
40. Burström G, Nachabe R, Homan R, Hoppenbrouwers J, Holthuizen R, Persson O, et al. Frameless patient tracking with adhesive optical skin markers for augmented reality surgical navigation in spine surgery. Spine. 2020;45(22):1598–604.
41. Drouin S, Kochanowska A, Kersten-Oertel M, Gerard IJ, Zelmann R, De Nigris D, et al. IBIS: an OR ready open-source platform for image-guided neurosurgery. Int J Comput Assist Radiol Surg. 2017;12(3):363–78.
42. Ewurum CH, Guo Y, Pagnha S, Feng Z, Luo X. Surgical navigation in orthopedics: workflow and system review. Int Orthop. 2018;1093:47–63.
43. Galletti B, Gazia F, Freni F, Sireci F, Galletti F. Endoscopic sinus surgery with and without computer assisted navigation: a retrospective study. Auris Nasus Larynx. 2019;46(4):520–5.
44. Mediavilla Guzmán A, Riad Deglow E, Zubizarreta-Macho Á, Agustín-Panadero R, Hernández MS. Accuracy of computer-aided dynamic navigation compared to computer-aided static navigation for dental implant placement: an in vitro study. J Clin Med. 2019;8(12):2123.

45. Majak M, Zuk M, Swiatek-Najwer E, Popek M, Pietruski P, editors. Biopsy procedure applied in MentorEye molecular surgical navigation system. European congress on computational methods in applied sciences and engineering. Springer; 2017.
46. Pelanis E, Teatini A, Eigl B, Regensburger A, Alzaga A, Kumar RP, et al. Evaluation of a novel navigation platform for laparoscopic liver surgery with organ deformation compensation using injected fiducials. Med Image Anal. 2021;69:101946.
47. Sukegawa S, Kanno T, Furuki Y. Application of computer-assisted navigation systems in oral and maxillofacial surgery. Jpn Dent Sci Rev. 2018;54(3):139–49.
48. Kurozumi K, Kameda M, Ishida J, Date I. Simultaneous combination of electromagnetic navigation with visual evoked potential in endoscopic transsphenoidal surgery: clinical experience and technical considerations. Acta Neurochir. 2017;159(6):1043.
49. Lavasani SN, Farnia P, Najafzadeh E, Saghatchi S, Samavati M, Abtahi H, et al. Bronchoscope motion tracking using centerline-guided Gaussian mixture model in navigated bronchoscopy. Phys Med Biol. 2021;66(2):025001.
50. Rania A, May I, Othman M. Evaluation of surgical-navigation system in management of orbital disorders. Med J Cairo Univ. 2019;87(June):1349–55.
51. Keeble H, Lavrador JP, Pereira N, Lente K, Brogna C, Gullan R, et al. Electromagnetic navigation systems and intraoperative neuromonitoring: reliability and feasibility study. Oper Neurosurg (Hagerstown). 2021;20(4):373–82.
52. Jaeger HA, Nardelli P, O'shea C, Tugwell J, Khan KA, Power T, et al. Automated catheter navigation with electromagnetic image guidance. IEEE Trans Biomed Eng. 2017;64(8):1972–9.
53. Maier J, Weiherer M, Huber M, Palm C. Optically tracked and 3D printed haptic phantom hand for surgical training system. Quant Imaging Med Surg. 2020;10(2):340.
54. Maier-Hein L, Franz A, Meinzer H-P, Wolf I, editors. Comparative assessment of optical tracking systems for soft tissue navigation with fiducial needles. Medical imaging 2008: visualization, image-guided procedures, and modeling. International Society for Optics and Photonics; 2008.
55. Marinetto E, Garcia-Mato D, Garcia A, Martinez S, Desco M, Pascau J. Multicamera optical tracker assessment for computer aided surgery applications. IEEE Access. 2018;6:64359–70.
56. Preim B, Botha CP. Visual computing for medicine: theory, algorithms, and applications. Boston: Newnes; 2013.
57. Attivissimo F, Lanzolla AML, Carlone S, Larizza P, Brunetti G. A novel electromagnetic tracking system for surgery navigation. Comput Assist Surg. 2018;23(1):42–52.
58. Navaei Lavasani S, Deevband M, Farnia P, Ahmadian A, Saghatchi S. Compensation of dynamic electromagnetic field distortion using simultaneous localization and mapping method with application in endobronchial ultrasound-transbronchial needle aspiration (EBUS-TBNA) guidance. Int J Med Robot. 2020;16(1):e2035.
59. Sadjadi H, Hashtrudi-Zaad K, Fichtinger G. Simultaneous localization and calibration for electromagnetic tracking systems. Int J Med Robot. 2016;12(2):189–98.
60. Wang J, Zhang W, Chen M. A survey of 3D image navigation and high precision dynamic registration in minimally invasive surgery. Procedia Comput Sci. 2018;131:320–6.
61. Maintz JA, Viergever MA. A survey of medical image registration. Med Image Anal. 1998;2(1):1–36.
62. Al-Azzawi N, Abdullah WAKW. MRI monomodal feature-based registration based on the efficiency of multiresolution representation and mutual information. Am J Biomed Eng. 2012;2(3):98–104.
63. Toth D, Miao S, Kurzendorfer T, Rinaldi CA, Liao R, Mansi T, et al. 3D/2D model-to-image registration by imitation learning for cardiac procedures. Int J Comput Assist Radiol Surg. 2018;13(8):1141–9.
64. Farnia P, Makkiabadi B, Ahmadian A, Alirezaie J, editors. Curvelet based residual complexity objective function for non-rigid registration of pre-operative MRI with intra-operative ultrasound images. 2016 38th annual international conference of the IEEE engineering in medicine and biology society (EMBC). IEEE; 2016.

65. Ahmadian A, Fathi Kazerooni A, Mohagheghi S, Amini Khoiy K, Sadr Hosseini M. A region-based anatomical landmark configuration for sinus surgery using image guided navigation system: a phantom-study. J Cranio-Maxillofac Surg. 2014;42(6):816–24.
66. Farnia P, Najafzadeh E, Ahmadian A, Makkiabadi B, Alimohamadi M, Alirezaie J, editors. Co-sparse analysis model based image registration to compensate brain shift by using intra-operative ultrasound imaging. 2018 40th annual international conference of the IEEE engineering in medicine and biology society (EMBC). IEEE; 2018.
67. Besl PJ, ND MK, editors. Method for registration of 3-D shapes. Sensor fusion IV: control paradigms and data structures. International Society for Optics and Photonics; 1992.
68. Farnia P, Ahmadian A, Khoshnevisan A, Jaberzadeh A, Serej ND, Kazerooni AF, editors. An efficient point based registration of intra-operative ultrasound images with MR images for computation of brain shift; a phantom study. 2011 annual international conference of the IEEE engineering in medicine and biology society. IEEE; 2011.
69. Noori SMR, Farnia P, Bayat M, Bahrami N, Shakourirad A, Ahmadian A. Automatic detection of symmetry plane for computer-aided surgical simulation in craniomaxillofacial surgery. Phys Eng Sci Med. 2020;43(3):1087–99.
70. Saghatchi S, Sadeghi MJ, Ahmadian A, Farahmand F, Sarkar S. Navigating an imaging instrument in a branched structure. Google Patents; 2018.
71. Ershad M, Ahmadian A, Dadashi Serej N, Saberi H, Amini KK. Minimization of target registration error for vertebra in image-guided spine surgery. Int J Comput Assist Radiol Surg. 2014;9(1):29–38.
72. Mohagheghi S, Ahmadian A, Yaghoobee S. Accuracy assessment of a marker-free method for registration of CT and stereo images applied in image-guided implantology: a phantom study. J Craniomaxillofac Surg. 2014;42(8):1977–84.
73. Lin Q, Cai K, Yang R, Xiao W, Huang J, Zhan Y, et al. Geometric calibration of markerless optical surgical navigation system. Int J Med Robot. 2019;15(2):e1978.
74. Serej ND, Ahmadian A, Mohagheghi S, Sadrehosseini SM. A projected landmark method for reduction of registration error in image-guided surgery systems. Int J Comput Assist Radiol Surg. 2015;10(5):541–54.
75. Raabe A, Krishnan R, Wolff R, Hermann E, Zimmermann M, Seifert V. Laser surface scanning for patient registration in intracranial image-guided surgery. Neurosurgery. 2002;50(4):797–803.
76. Wang D, Ma D, Wong ML, Wáng YXJ. Recent advances in surgical planning & navigation for tumor biopsy and resection. Quant Imaging Med Surg. 2015;5(5):640.
77. Knoops PG, Beaumont CA, Borghi A, Rodriguez-Florez N, Breakey RW, Rodgers W, et al. Comparison of three-dimensional scanner systems for craniomaxillofacial imaging. J Plast Reconstr Aesthet Surg. 2017;70(4):441–9.
78. Zheng Y, Doermann D. Robust point matching for nonrigid shapes by preserving local neighborhood structures. IEEE Trans Pattern Anal Mach Intell. 2006;28(4):643–9.
79. Jian B, Vemuri BC. Robust point set registration using gaussian mixture models. IEEE Trans Pattern Anal Mach Intell. 2010;33(8):1633–45.
80. Myronenko A, Song X. Point set registration: coherent point drift. IEEE Trans Pattern Anal Mach Intell. 2010;32(12):2262–75.
81. Mohammadi A, Ahmadian A, Rabbani S, Fattahi E, Shirani S. A combined registration and finite element analysis method for fast estimation of intraoperative brain shift; phantom and animal model study. Int J Med Robot. 2017;13(4):e1792.
82. Mohammadi A, Ahmadian A, Azar AD, Sheykh AD, Amiri F, Alirezaie J. Estimation of intraoperative brain shift by combination of stereovision and doppler ultrasound: phantom and animal model study. Int J Comput Assist Radiol Surg. 2015;10(11):1753–64.
83. Gerard IJ, Kersten-Oertel M, Petrecca K, Sirhan D, Hall JA, Collins DL. Brain shift in neuronavigation of brain tumors: a review. Med Image Anal. 2017;35:403–20.
84. Bayer S, Maier A, Ostermeier M, Fahrig R. Intraoperative imaging modalities and compensation for brain shift in tumor resection surgery. Int J Biomed Imaging. 2017;2017:6028645.

85. Kuhnt D, Bauer MH, Nimsky C. Brain shift compensation and neurosurgical image fusion using intraoperative MRI: current status and future challenges. Crit Rev Biomed Eng. 2012;40(3):175–85.
86. Farnia P, Ahmadian A, Shabanian T, Serej ND, Alirezaie J. Brain-shift compensation by non-rigid registration of intra-operative ultrasound images with preoperative MR images based on residual complexity. Int J Comput Assist Radiol Surg. 2015;10(5):555–62.
87. Stummer W, Molina ES. Fluorescence imaging/agents in tumor resection. Neurosurg Clin. 2017;28(4):569–83.
88. Mehrmohammadi M, Joon Yoon S, Yeager D, Emelianov Y, S. Photoacoustic imaging for cancer detection and staging. Curr Mol Imaging. 2013;2(1):89–105.
89. Najafzadeh E, Ghadiri H, Alimohamadi M, Farnia P, Mehrmohammadi M, Ahmadian A. Application of multi-wavelength technique for photoacoustic imaging to delineate tumor margins during maximum-safe resection of glioma: a preliminary simulation study. J Clin Neurosci. 2019;70:242–6.
90. Najafzadeh E, Ghadiri H, Alimohamadi M, Farnia P, Mehrmohammadi M, Ahmadian A. Evaluation of multi-wavelengths LED-based photoacoustic imaging for maximum safe resection of glioma: a proof of concept study. Int J Comput Assist Radiol Surg. 2020;15:1053–62.
91. Arabpou S, Najafzadeh E, Farnia P, Ahmadian A, Ghadiri H, Akhoundi MSA. Detection of early stages dental caries using photoacoustic signals: the simulation study. Front Biomed Technol. 2019.
92. Jokerst J, Moore C, Hariri A. Photoacoustic imaging for noninvasive periodontal probing depth measurements. Google Patents; 2021.
93. Yan Y, John S, Ghalehnovi M, Kabbani L, Kennedy NA, Mehrmohammadi M. Photoacoustic imaging for image-guided endovenous laser ablation procedures. Sci Rep. 2019;9(1):1–10.
94. Eddins B, Bell MAL. Design of a multifiber light delivery system for photoacoustic-guided surgery. J Biomed Opt. 2017;22(4):041011.
95. Wang LV. Photoacoustic imaging and spectroscopy. CRC press; 2017.
96. Najafzadeh E, Farnia P, Ahmadian A, Ghadiri H. Light-emitting diode based photoacoustic imaging system. Front Biomed Technol. 2020;7(3):200–4.
97. Beard P. Biomedical photoacoustic imaging. Interface focus. 2011;1(4):602–31.
98. Zackrisson S, Van De Ven S, Gambhir S. Light in and sound out: emerging translational strategies for photoacoustic imaging. Cancer Res. 2014;74(4):979–1004.
99. Farnia P, Mohammadi M, Najafzadeh E, Alimohamadi M, Makkiabadi B, Ahmadian AJBP, et al. High-quality photoacoustic image reconstruction based on deep convolutional neural network: towards intra-operative photoacoustic imaging. Biomed Phys Eng Express. 2020;6(4):045019.
100. Farnia P, Makkiabadi B, Alimohamadi M, Najafzadeh E, Basij M, Yan Y, et al. Photoacoustic-MR image registration based on a co-sparse analysis model to compensate for brain shift. Sensors (Basel, Switzerland) 2022;22(6).
101. Farnia P, Najafzadeh E, Hariri A, Lavasani SN, Makkiabadi B, Ahmadian A, et al. Dictionary learning technique enhances signal in LED-based photoacoustic imaging. Biomed Opt Express. 2020;11(5):2533–47.
102. Najafzadeh E, Farnia P, Lavasani SN, Basij M, Yan Y, Ghadiri H, et al. Photoacoustic image improvement based on a combination of sparse coding and filtering. J Biomed Opt. 2020;25(10):106001.
103. Hasan W, Daly MJ, Chan HHL, Qiu J, Irish JCJTL. Intraoperative cone-beam CT-guided osteotomy navigation in mandible and maxilla surgery. Laryngoscope. 2020;130(5):1166–72.
104. Marescaux J, Diana M. Next step in minimally invasive surgery: hybrid image-guided surgery. J Pediatr Surg. 2015;50(1):30–6.
105. Cutolo F. Augmented reality in image-guided surgery. 2019.

106. Lungu AJ, Swinkels W, Claesen L, Tu P, Egger J, Chen X. A review on the applications of virtual reality, augmented reality and mixed reality in surgical simulation: an extension to different kinds of surgery. Expert Rev Med Devices. 2021;18(1):47–62.
107. McKnight RR, Pean CA, Buck JS, Hwang JS, Hsu JR, Pierrie SN. Virtual reality and augmented reality—translating surgical training into surgical technique. Curr Rev Musculoskelet Med. 2020;13:663–74.
108. Liu K, Gao Y, Abdelrehem A, Zhang L, Chen X, Xie L, et al. Augmented reality navigation method for recontouring surgery of craniofacial fibrous dysplasia. Sci Rep. 2021;11(1):1–7.
109. Aziz MJ, Zade AAT, Farnia P, Alimohamadi M, Makkiabadi B, Ahmadian A, Alirezaie J. Accurate automatic glioma segmentation in brain MRI images based on CapsNet. 2021 43rd Annual International Conference of the IEEE Engineering in Medicine & Biology Society (EMBC): IEEE; 2021. p. 3882–5.
110. Gholizadeh-Ansari M, Alirezaie J, Babyn P. Deep learning for low-dose CT denoising using perceptual loss and edge detection layer. J Digit Imaging. 2020;33:504–15.
111. Rivas-Blanco I, Pérez-Del-Pulgar CJ, García-Morales I, Muñoz VF. A review on deep learning in minimally invasive surgery. IEEE Access. 2021;9:48658–78.
112. Diana M, Marescaux J. Robotic surgery. J Br Surg. 2015;102(2):e15–28.
113. Gimenez ME. Percutaneous image-guided surgery. Int J Gastrointest Intervent. 2019;8(1):2–5.

Navigation in Orthognathic Surgery

Constantinus Politis, Yi Sun, Tian Lei, and Eman Shaheen

1 Introduction

Plath et al. reported about 30 orthognathic patients being operated since 1996 using intraoperative navigation for positioning the maxilla intraoperatively in Le Fort I and bimaxillary orthognathic surgery cases [1]. They used navigation simultaneously with intraoperative splints to check the jaw position. In fact it was rather used as a measuring device than a guiding device of the maxilla toward the correct position. This remains to be the case in 2021 despite many attempts to evolve to splintless orthognathic surgery [2]. Rather than routine use in orthognathic surgery, most surgeons evaluate intraoperative navigation systems as a useful adjunct tool in the correction of complex facial malformations such as facial asymmetry [3, 4].

2 Orthognathic Surgery

Orthognathic surgical procedures as meant in this chapter aim to displace parts of the maxillo-facial skeleton into another position in space. Both linear and rotational movements in all dimensions are needed to correct maxillofacial deformities. In

C. Politis (✉) · Y. Sun · E. Shaheen
Oral and Maxillofacial Surgery—Imaging and Pathology Research Group, Department of Imaging and Pathology, University of Leuven, Leuven, Belgium

Department of Oral & Maxillofacial Surgery, University Hospitals Leuven, Leuven, Belgium
e-mail: Constantinus.politis@uzleuven.be

T. Lei
Department of oral and maxillofacial surgery, College of Stomatology, The Fourth Military Medical University, Xi'an, Shaanxi, China

S. A. Parhiz et al. (eds.), *Navigation in Oral and Maxillofacial Surgery*,
https://doi.org/10.1007/978-3-031-06223-0_2

daily practice, the most commonly used procedures are Le Fort I, sagittal split of the lower jaw and genioplasty osteotomies.

These surgical techniques exist for about 50 years or even longer. Le Fort I osteotomy aims at displacing the entire tooth bearing region of the upper jaw, while sagittal split osteotomy aims at displacing the entire tooth bearing region of the lower jaw and genioplasty allows only to displace the anterior lower border of the mandible with its internal muscular attachments.

The basics on which the planning of these procedures rely upon are still in widespread use. Planning relies on clinical examination of the patient, the definition of a patient's problem list, plaster casts of the occlusion, a wax-bite, a panoramic radiograph, a cephalometric analysis based on two-dimensional (2D) lateral cephalogram image of the maxillofacial skeleton.

With the introduction of computers, computer software, three-dimensional (3D) radiographic imaging techniques such as computer tomography (CT) or low-dose cone beam CT (CBCT), scanning of occlusion and low-cost 3D printers, much of the planning has been transferred into a 3D virtual environment, but without fundamentally changing the planning process.

The planning process is essentially different in mono-maxillary approach compared to bimaxillary approach. In mono-maxillary approach, the dental casts (physical or virtual) of the mobilized part are placed together with the opposite occlusion in the desired functional occlusion and fixed together as to allow a splint production (manual made or 3D printed) [5, 6]. Both 3D printed splints or conventionally manufactured with self-cured resin (acrylic) splint will position one jaw exactly the same way to the opposite occlusion since the transfer objective is the occlusion of teeth. The preoperative wax-bite does not play any role in mono-maxillary surgery.

In bimaxillary approach, the planning process is quite different and depends on the jaw mobilized first. If the upper jaw is to be mobilized first, then the upper jaw is to be positioned and fixed in a pre-planned position. This position can be determined in different ways: purely clinically, purely on cephalometric analysis (2D or 3D), based on software tools or a combination of these methods. Once in the operating theater, this predetermined position needs to be found and secured. Again the planning in the virtual space needs to be transferred into the real-life world.

Usually, in the traditional sequence, acetate overlay "templates" of the maxilla are moved on the existing tracing paper in the amount, inclination of occlusal plane and direction necessary to achieve the desired esthetic result. On the basis of anticipated changes in the hard tissues (bone + occlusion), a new soft tissue profile is traced assuming the hard-to-soft tissue ratio of changes is known.

The planned movements of the maxilla and maxillary teeth are now simulated on dental casts. A face bow transfer is used to mount the models on an adjustable articulator for proper orientation of the maxillary cast to the glenoid fossae and mandibular hinge axis. The models are mounted in centric relationship on a Dentatus articulator using the wax-bite. This articulator simulates the occlusion in the mouth according to the position of teeth registered with the wax-bite.

The setup is ready for surgery simulation using the articulator where the upper jaw is sectioned at a height above the apices, just as would be done intraoperatively. The mobilized part is moved according to the plan and fixed in the desired position in the articulator with sticky wax. The vertical, horizontal, and anteroposterior dimensional changes are recorded on the articulator and verified to match the planning. An inter-occlusal splint acrylic splint is created with self-cured resin and will allow to fixate the maxillary segments into the planned position opposite to the occlusion of the lower jaw [7].

The virtual workflow is in essence the same. The occlusion of upper and lower jaw is registered according to a digitized wax-bite. The dento-osseous segment of the upper jaw is segmented in order to allow autonomous movement of the segmented part out of the remaining virtual volume. A virtual inter-occlusal splint is constructed and 3D printed in biocompatible polymers with almost the same accuracy as a physical acrylic splint [6].

In the operating theater, with the maxilla and mandible in intermaxillary fixation, the mandible is held in the most retruded position possible and rotated until the occlusal margin of the upper incisor teeth reach a planned vertical position in the patient. If the vertical position mandates removal of obstructive bony interferences, these need to be removed. If the vertical position leaves a gap between the osteotomy lines, a bone graft may be needed.

The sticky wax to stabilize the dento-osseous segment in the articulator and the "save-in-the-new-position-function" in the software finds a surgical correlate in the tight intermaxillary fixation of the parts kept together on the interocclusal splint with manual pressure to ensure the vertical position with the condyle in its most retruded position. The retropositioned maxilla is then fixed with osteosynthesis plates.

Intermaxillary fixation is removed, and the lower jaw can be further treated following the mono-maxillary approach. If the lower jaw is to be mobilized first, the steps are in essence the same, but in reversed order. The preference to start bimaxillary surgery in the lower jaw or in the upper jaw is at the surgeon's discretion.

Understanding the difference between accuracy and precision is very important. Accuracy is choosing the right target, precision is hitting the chosen target (Fig. 1). Contemporary orthognathic surgery is not very accurate nor very precise for many reasons. Accuracy is lacking due to the fact that patient and referrer satisfaction with the end result cannot be translated into objective targets. Reaching correct occlusion is usually not the main concern, since the combined treatment of orthognathic surgery with orthodontics usually reaches an occlusal contact precision within 20–30 μm and an acceptable overbite and overjet within a few mm which is necessary to properly function. The dento-osseous fragments of the upper and lower jaws together in a correct occlusion can however be positioned in a larger number of degrees of freedom (typically six: including three translational and three rotational movements). These degrees of freedom are used to reach a pleasant soft tissue profile and an "en face" appearance, a pleasant incisal show both in rest (usually

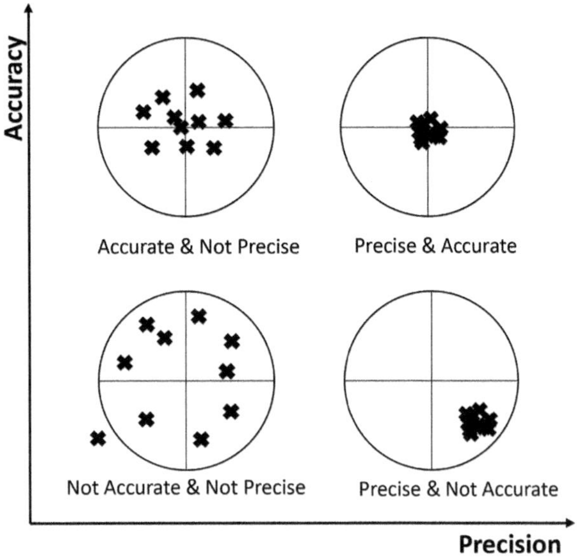

Fig. 1 Difference between accuracy and precision

between 2 and 4 mm) and while laughing, correct dental and skeletal midlines and absence of occlusal cants. Not only is this bandwidth mainly subjective and influenced by socio-cultural tastes, but also the ratio at which soft tissues follow hard tissues are not exactly determined for each point in the face, nor is the influence on the nose exactly predictable. The subjective result will be influenced by numerous adjunctive procedures possible (soft tissue augmentation, soft tissue reduction, hard tissue augmentation, cosmetic lip procedures, face lift, Botox, rhinoplasty). Cultural differences very often include a different appreciation concerning the flatness of the upper jaw, the amount of incisor shown in resting position, the amount of gummy smile, the width of the nose, and the prominence of the cheeks and zygomatic areas.

Once a target position of the upper jaw is chosen within the bandwidth, which hopefully will please the patient (accuracy), the next goal is to achieve precision for both the occlusion and the planned position of the upper jaw. The final occlusion can always be reached using a final splint which precisely fits both occlusal surfaces. Once rigid fixation with manually adapted stock osteosynthesis plates is applied, intermaxillary fixation is removed and occlusion can be checked. If necessary, rigid fixation can be re-applied to ascertain the desired occlusion.

As to the precision of the upper jaw, the surgeon has to rely on the intermediate splint and intraoperative measurements on the patient to ascertain the correct position of the upper jaw. The resulting difference between preoperative planning and achieved results varies with the magnitude of displacement and direction of displacement. Large individual differences between patients are noticed [7, 8].

Precision of bimaxillary surgery is affected by accumulated errors starting from the intermediate splint, the existing joint play in the temporomandibular joint, measurements of the repositioned upper jaw in 3D space, and errors induced by the fixation appliances of the upper jaw.

Errors in the intermediate splint have been extensively reviewed, and the main contributors are errors in wax-bite [9] and errors in mock surgery of the mounted plaster casts in the articulator in case of conventional planning.

The joint play in the temporomandibular joint refers to the difference between the condylar position used during the planning process and the condylar position during general anesthesia with the patient in supine position under general relaxation and the proximal fragment manually repositioned in its presumably most posterior position in the fossa.

Fixation appliance errors relate to nonpassive bending of osteosynthesis plates, eccentric drilling and possibly uneven distribution of plates.

Errors in measurements of the repositioned upper jaw in 3D space are serious and technically unsolved. Both internal reference points (IRP) and external reference points (ERP) are used. IRP are arbitrarily chosen landmarks on the bone above and below Le Fort I osteotomy cuts on the lateral maxillary walls for intraoperative positioning of the maxilla. ERP are intraoperative positioning points based on the soft tissue nasion (N′) or hard tissue nasion (N) by inserting a reference screw at N (Fig. 2).

Scatterplots of horizontal and vertical measurements of dental landmarks comparing preoperative planning and postoperative outcome show that the target is often missed for several mm both as under- or over-correction [7, 8]. This indicates that the splint-based repositioning technique often fails as reliable guide for horizontal displacements and that the IRP and ERP do function as a reliable aid to position the incisor margin but fail to vertically reach targets in the molar area of the maxilla.

To overcome these errors, one should rely on a splint-less technique in which the maxillary volume as a whole can be displaced to the target location with haptic and auditory control once the entire volume has reached the exact target location and is in “freeze” in that location until rigid fixation is applied.

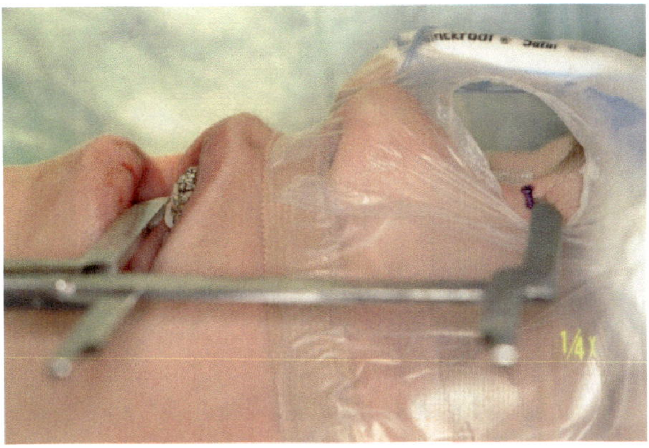

Fig. 2 The caliper measures the distance between a screw inserted at nasion and the incisal edge of the upper incisor

3 Navigation in Orthognathic Surgery

Image-guided surgery (i.e., navigation) consists of four main components: preoperative 3D images, computer, tracking system, and an instrument or pointer used by the surgeon [10]. The preoperative images could be magnetic resonance imaging (MRI), positron emission tomography (PET), CT, or CBCT. However, for orthognathic surgery, CT and CBCT are the most commonly used images. One frequently used navigation system in orthognathic surgery is presented in Fig. 3 (Kolibri System, Brainlab, Munich, Germany) [11, 12]. The navigation system is equipped with a camera system with infrared light (tracking system, Fig. 3a), a navigation star which is a skull reference base fixated at the head of the patient (Figs. 3b and 4a) and a pointer (surgeon's instrument, Figs. 3c and 4a). The preoperative CT/CBCT is imported into the navigation software then the surgeon registers the preoperative CT/CBCT image using landmarks [11] or surface registration [12] by means of the pointer to link the patient images to the computer screen with the pointer. After registration, the pointer becomes visible on the computer screen as shown in Fig. 4b, c. Whenever the pointer is applied on the patient within the visible reach of the infrared sensor, the pointer will appear on the preoperative CT/CBCT scan.

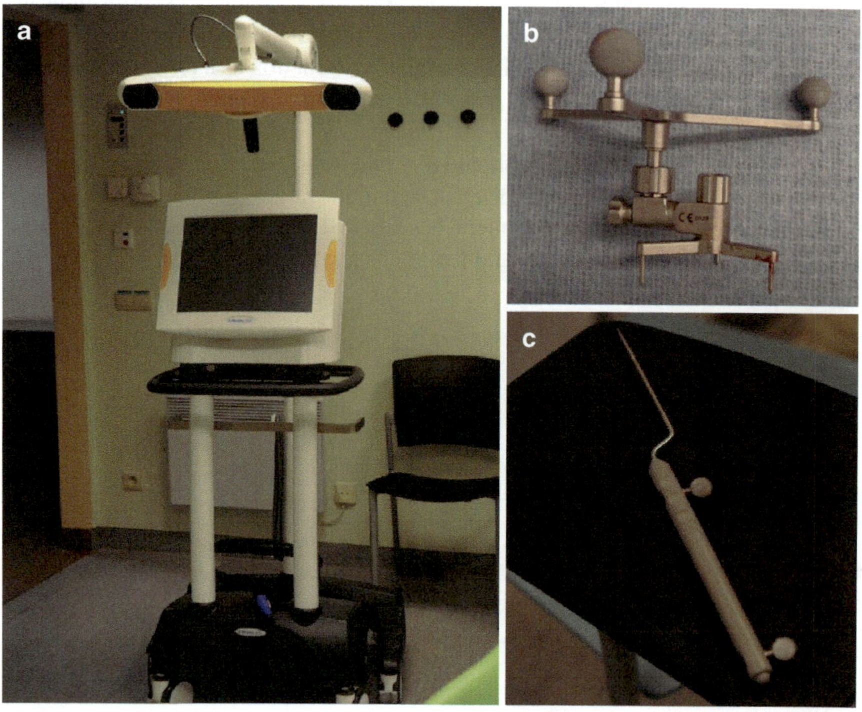

Fig. 3 An example of navigation system used during orthognathic surgery (Kolibri System, Brainlab, Munich, Germany). (**a**) The navigation system consisting of a camera with infrared light. (**b**) The skull reference base (navigation star). (**c**) The pointer

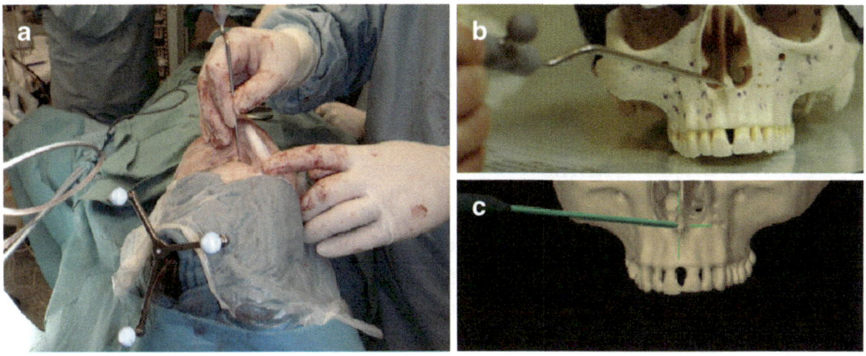

Fig. 4 Navigation system setup. (**a**) Registration step using the pointer. (**b**) Physical pointer becomes visible virtually on the computer screen (**c**)

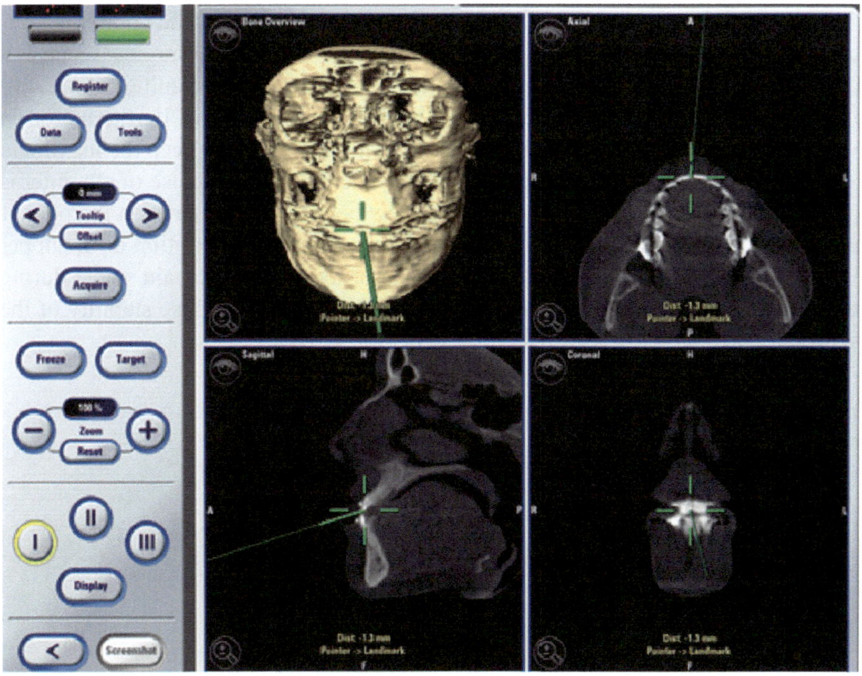

Fig. 5 Surgical movement maxilla using navigation system on preoperative CBCT image. In the sagittal direction, the pointer is physically positioned at the edge of the dental midline of the central incisors. The axis of the pointer is then positioned parallel to the FHP. Coming from the green cross, which represented the pointer tip showed no deviation in the midline

Navigation is about precision, not accuracy. To evaluate the positioning of the maxilla, the pointer needs to be directed either parallel to the Frankfurter Horizontal Plane (FHP) for horizontal measurements or perpendicular to FHP for vertical measurements on a specific point to evaluate the deviation from that point (Fig. 5).

Most measurements occur at the level of incisors since posterior measurements of a maxilla in intermaxillary fixation is rather challenging [12].

4 Unaccounted Claims

Navigation systems claim to have enabled surgeons to avoid injuring important anatomic structures due to the real-time visualization of the accurate position of surgical instruments; however, these claims are not supported by evidence [13].

5 Limitations

To date, no such navigation system exists. The position sensor of the pointer in optical surgical navigation is only a tool that allows to measure the surgical change at certain points and mainly anterior points (incisors) due to the difficulties of measuring points posteriorly on the maxilla in intermaxillary fixation. Furthermore, no volumetric evaluation is allowed, let alone that it could guide or keep the maxilla in a "freeze" position once the target is reached. The intraoperative use of a pointer is not intuitive and requires an unobstructed view between the spheres on the pointer and the infrared light of the camera. The landmark-based registration of the upper jaw is at best "clinically acceptable." The star array needs to remain stable during the entire surgical procedure since a screw failure will lead to lose stability of the skull reference base and thus the entire system (Fig. 6).

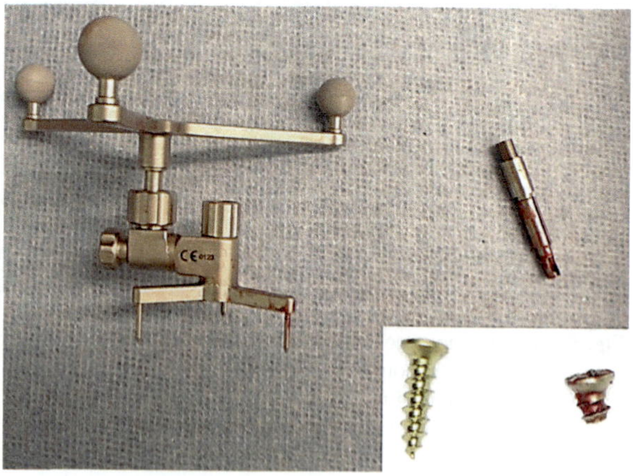

Fig. 6 Screw failure leads to loss of stability of the skull reference base and the entire system

6 Future Prospects

Improvements are required where a tracking device should be mounted on the dento-osseous part with sufficient fiducial markers to allow spatial registration of the entire dento-osseous volume, without impeding surgery [14]. This does not solve the needed "freeze" in the desired target position, necessary to stabilize and definitely assure that position. This would require simultaneous robotic intervention fed with navigational data. This has been shown to work successfully but only in laboratory conditions [15].

The same limitations apply to augmented reality tools where the loosened dento-osseous part of the maxilla is visually tracked in superposition with volume rendered CT. These systems still need intraoperative splints and do not allow stabilization of the translocated part in the target position [16, 17].

Rather than "push" the loosened dento-osseous segment of the maxilla into the target position, one could imagine to "pull" the dento-osseous segment into the final position. This requires 3D printed patient-specific osteosynthesis plates (PSP) which perfectly fit to the underlying bone and are rigid (Titanium Grade 2). PSP can serve as skeletally supported templates and at the same time allow to stabilize the maxilla in all dimensions [18, 19]. This solution does exist, but unfortunately costly and allows no margin for error nor any intraoperative adaptability, let alone that bony interferences hampering to reach the end position could be visualized intraoperatively. Point-of-care titanium printing facilities in hospital settings could address cost–benefit issues.

7 Conclusions

Since their introduction in 1996, image-guided navigation systems in orthognathic surgery have failed to live up to the promise of splint-less orthognathic surgery, mainly due to the absence of tracking tools which allow to visualize the loosened dento-osseous segment of the jaw, together with the absence of tools to "freeze" the maxilla in the target position.

References

1. Plath T, Hoffmeister B, Neumann P, Siebert D, Tolxdorff T, Wolff K, et al. Positioning of the maxilla in orthognathic surgery using intraoperative navigation. Int J Oral Maxillofac Surg. 1999;28:62. https://doi.org/10.1016/S0901-5027(99)80839-X.
2. Tanaka M, Sato H, Inada T, Yaso A, Ogura H, Shirota T. Maxillary repositioning using a CAD/CAM wafer and an intraoperative navigation system for bimaxillary orthognathic sur-

gery using segmental Le fort I osteotomy: a pilot study. J Oral Maxillofac Surg Med Pathol. 2021;33(6):581–6. https://doi.org/10.1016/j.ajoms.2021.04.003.
3. Bell RB. Computer planning and intraoperative navigation in orthognathic surgery. J Oral Maxillofac Surg. 2011;69(3):592–605. https://doi.org/10.1016/j.joms.2009.06.030.
4. Azarmehr I, Stokbro K, Bell RB, Thygesen T. Surgical navigation: a systematic review of indications, treatments, and outcomes in oral and maxillofacial surgery. J Oral Maxillofac Surg. 2017;75(9):1987–2005. https://doi.org/10.1016/j.joms.2017.01.004.
5. Shaheen E, Sun Y, Jacobs R, Politis C. Three-dimensional printed final occlusal splint for orthognathic surgery: design and validation. Int J Oral Maxillofac Surg. 2017;46(1):67–71.
6. Shaheen E, Coopman R, Jacobs R, Politis C. Optimized 3D virtually planned intermediate splints for bimaxillary orthognathic surgery: a clinical validation study in 20 patients. J Craniomaxillofacial Surg. 2018;46(9):1441–7. https://doi.org/10.1016/j.jcms.2018.05.050.
7. Govaerts D, Shaheen E, Coopman R, De Mol A, Sun Y, Politis C. Accuracy of Le Fort I osteotomy in bimaxillary splint-based orthognathic surgery: focus on posterior maxillary movements. Int J Oral Maxillofac Surg. 2018;47(11):1398–404. https://doi.org/10.1016/j.ijom.2018.05.008.
8. Mulier D, Shaheen E, Shujaat S, Fieuws S, Jacobs R, Politis C. How accurate is digital-assisted Le Fort I maxillary osteotomy? A three-dimensional perspective. Int J Oral Maxillofac Surg. 2020;49(1):69–74.
9. Agbaje JO, Sun Y, Lambrichts I, Politis C. Problems during orthognathic surgery resulting from errors in diagnostic wax bite. J Craniofac Surg. 2013;24(3):999–1001. http://www.ncbi.nlm.nih.gov/pubmed/23714932
10. Nijmeh AD, Goodger NM, Hawkes D, Edwards PJ, McGurk M. Image-guided navigation in oral and maxillofacial surgery. Br J Oral Maxillofac Surg. 2005;43(4):294–302.
11. Sun Y, Luebbers HT, Agbaje JO, Schepers S, Vrielinck L, Lambrichts I, et al. Validation of anatomical landmarks-based registration for image-guided surgery: an in-vitro study. J Craniomaxillofacial Surg. 2013;41(6):522–6. https://doi.org/10.1016/j.jcms.2012.11.017.
12. Sun Y, Luebbers HT, Agbaje JO, Lambrichts I, Politis C. The accuracy of image-guided navigation for maxillary positioning in bimaxillary surgery. J Craniofac Surg. 2014;25(3):1095–9.
13. Shim BK, Shin HS, Nam SM, Kim YB. Real-time navigation-assisted orthognathic surgery. J Craniofac Surg. 2013;24(1):221–5.
14. Chen X, Li Y, Xu L, Sun Y, Politis C, Jiang X. A real time image-guided reposition system for the loosed bone graft in orthognathic surgery. Comput Assist Surg (Abingdon). 2021;26(1):1–8.
15. Han JJ, Woo S-Y, Yi W-J, Hwang SJ. Robot-assisted maxillary positioning in orthognathic surgery: a feasibility and accuracy evaluation. J Clin Med. 2021;10(12):2596.
16. Mischkowski RA, Zinser MJ, Kübler AC, Krug B, Seifert U, Zöller JE. Application of an augmented reality tool for maxillary positioning in orthognathic surgery - a feasibility study. J Craniomaxillofacial Surg. 2006;34(8):478–83.
17. Wagner A, Rasse M, Millesi W, Ewers R. Virtual reality for orthognathic surgery: the augmented reality environment concept. J Oral Maxillofac Surg. 1997;55(5):456–62.
18. Stokbro K, Borg SW, Andersen MØ, Thygesen T. Patient-specific 3D printed plates improve stability of Le Fort 1 osteotomies in vitro. J Craniomaxillofacial Surg. 2019;47(3):394–9.
19. Stokbro K, Bell RB, Thygesen T. Patient-specific printed plates improve surgical accuracy in vitro. J Oral Maxillofac Surg. 2018;76(12):2647.e1–9. https://doi.org/10.1016/j.joms.2018.08.002.

Navigation in Trauma Surgery

Likith Reddy, Cesar Rivera, and Ritesh Bhattacharjee

1 Introduction

Intraoperative navigation is a system that was originally employed in the use of neurosurgery. The use of this technology was later redefined and polished to where other specialties incorporated it into their uses. In a brief definition, "navigation means a device that can accurately locate critical anatomical structures, the safest way to reach that target, and the orientation around which safe and reliable surgery can be carried out" [1]. This has been utilized as a reliable tool for real-time analysis of maxillofacial structures as compared to preoperative scans as well as allowing for structures that are usually not visualized during surgery.

Surgery in the maxillofacial region has been performed to reestablish function, facial symmetry, and projection to bring about esthetic harmony. In the setting of trauma, the main purpose is to restore function and cosmesis that has been altered due to the traumatic event, obtaining a result that matches the pretraumatic state. Surgeons have relied in different imaging modalities to diagnose, plan, and execute such surgeries. Despite the notable success, there are still areas in which the current state of imaging modalities has limitations, leading to issues when reestablishing

L. Reddy (✉)
Department of Oral & Maxillofacial Surgery, College of Dentistry, Texas A&M University, Dallas, TX, USA

Oral & Maxillofacial Surgery, Baylor University Medical Center, Dallas, TX, USA

Medical Education, College of Medicine, Texas A& M University, Dallas, TX, USA
e-mail: lreddy@tamu.edu

C. Rivera · R. Bhattacharjee
Department of Oral & Maxillofacial Surgery, College of Dentistry, Texas A&M University, Dallas, TX, USA

Oral & Maxillofacial Surgery, Baylor University Medical Center, Dallas, TX, USA

S. A. Parhiz et al. (eds.), *Navigation in Oral and Maxillofacial Surgery*,
https://doi.org/10.1007/978-3-031-06223-0_3

the proper projections of the face. Most of these problems arise due to the difficulty assessing, intraoperatively, the symmetry of corrected or repositioned hard tissue, orbital contours, especially in the posterior aspects, missing segments that need to be reconstructed, and all the variability those changes lead to in the different planes three-dimensionally.

The implementation of intraoperative navigation in maxillofacial trauma has been used in the past with good outcomes. The application of navigation in the realm of facial trauma has established in orbital fractures, zygomaticomaxillary fractures (ZMC), removal of foreign bodies, maxillomandibular reconstruction, gun-shot injuries, and others. Navigation has allowed for a better symmetrical component when using the uninjured contralateral site as a template, especially when reinstating projections and contours (Fig. 1). In addition, navigation allows for visualization of fracture reduction in planes that are hard to visualize. There is also situational awareness. This property of navigation allows the operator to better identify nearby structures, locate in a three-dimensional plane, and avoid damage to specific structures in the range of millimeters.

Recent studies have been performed to evaluate the usage of intraoperative navigation as compared to other imaging modalities. In 2015, the position of implants in 10 cadaver heads (20 orbits) was analyzed using navigation and no navigation. Dubois et al. found that "the consistency of orbital reconstruction was lower in the traditional reconstructions than in the navigation group in the parameters of translation and rotation. Implant position also differed significantly in the parameters of translation and rotation" [2]. They concluded that navigation provides a more predictable result in reconstruction of orbital injuries as well as improving position of orbital implants. In addition, Xi Gong et al. [3] evaluated the outcomes of delayed surgery in ZMC fractures with and without navigation. They found that absolute difference bilaterally in malar eminence was significantly lower in the navigation

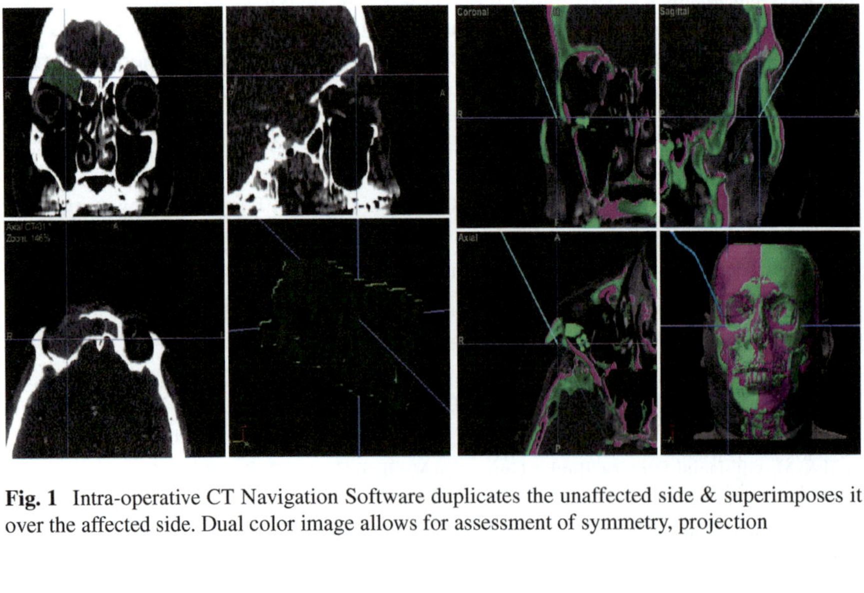

Fig. 1 Intra-operative CT Navigation Software duplicates the unaffected side & superimposes it over the affected side. Dual color image allows for assessment of symmetry, projection

group. The percentage of patient with <2 mm of difference between both ZMC eminence and width was 79% in the navigation group, while in the non-navigation group was 35.9%. The usefulness of intraoperative navigation has been tested and proven to be a useful tool in maxillofacial trauma. This chapter will go over those specific applications in the different types of trauma to the different areas of the maxillofacial complex.

2 Application of Navigation in Zygomaticomaxillary Complex Fractures

Zygomaticomaxillary complex (ZMC) is a key component of the midface that determines midfacial protrusion, width as well as contributing to the orbital floor and rim, maintaining eye position and participating in ocular projection. ZMC fractures can lead to obvious cosmetic defects in the face, functional deficits if interfering with mouth function, visual disturbances if orbit damaged, among others. Traditionally, operative treatment of ZMC fractures have been with open reduction and internal fixation when there is a functional or esthetic compromise. The approach to the fractures depends on the fracture pattern and/or the displacement of the fractures. The verification of reduction intraoperatively has been performed with direct visualization, as well as direct visualization of soft tissues for esthetic results.

These fractures are complex to repair and are difficult to master. The appropriate reduction of fractures, in addition to the adequate restoration of bony contours, is critical to reestablish cosmesis and function. Three dimensionally, ZMC fractures can be hard to reposition into an anatomical correct location. Proper alignment of the zygomaticosphenoid (ZS) suture is key for reduction of ZMC fractures. Most ZMC fractures generally have medial rotation of the displaced segment with loss of anterior-posterior projection. It is paramount to correct this 3D distortion by the correct alignment of the zygoma relative to the cranial base. This alignment can be challenging, especially in cases where there is comminution of any of the component of the ZMC tetrapod. Intraoperative navigation allows for real-time analysis of the reduction of the ZS as well as the other components of the tetrapod (Fig. 2).

Multiple authors have described the usage of navigation in ZMC fractures successfully, finding an increased accuracy in reductions. Zhang et al. [4] reported 20 cases of unilateral ZMC fractures finding that the group where navigation was used had significant better reductions than the control group. They found that in the experimental group the average distance from the bony landmarks was 0.59 mm, while in the control group was 1.23, suggesting that the postoperative reduction in the navigation group was closer to ideal than the one in the control group.

Different techniques have been utilized for the evaluation of reduction. Ogino et al. [5] reported two approaches for this. On the one hand, they use the mirroring technique to compare the reduction based on the contralateral and unaffected side. This was used as a guide to measure face projections. On the other hand, they used

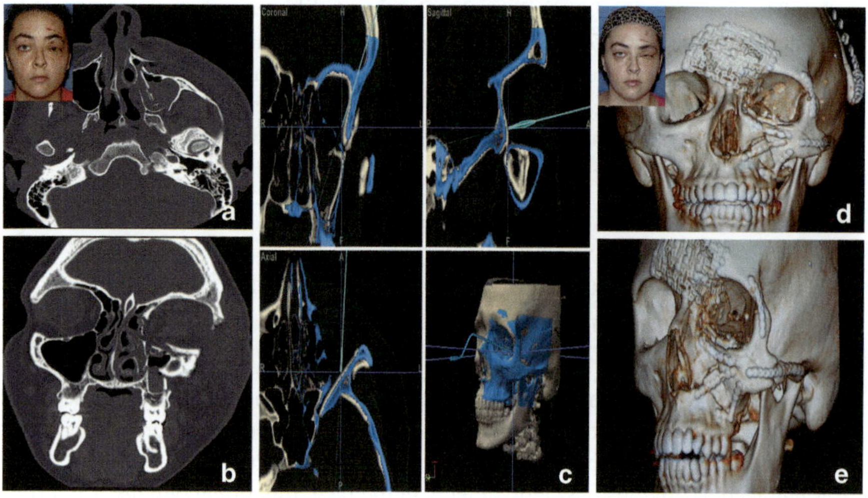

Fig. 2 Application of navigation in zygomaticomaxillary fracture reconstruction, (**a**, **b**) Pre-op CT imaging (**c**) Intra-op navigation for real time zygomatic suture reduction (**d**, **e**) Post-op 3D reconstruction

probes to evaluate the mean distances from the midline of the face. Midline of face was based on anterior and posterior nasal spine. Once this is established, the distance between the midline and the zygomatic arch was obtained in both affected and unaffected site. This was then compared after reduction. They found that both the techniques are adequate for as tools in ZMC fractures.

To a more elemental function, navigation can be used for the reduction of zygomatic arch when fixation is not needed. In these fractures, there is usually a depression noted and palpated just anterior to the tragus with possible trismus depending upon impingement with the coronoid process. Vestibular approach or Gillies method can be used for exposure, and the election of the preferred flat elevator can be used for reduction. Generally, this technique relies on visualization of soft tissues projection, tactile analysis during reduction as well as listening to the click of bone during reduction. Intraoperative navigation can be further used to appreciate the actual bony reduction in these cases. Even in times where there is soft tissue edema, reduction of the fractures can be observed by real-time feedback. Mirroring technique can also be used to evaluate for bilateral symmetry and changes can be made if needed.

In displaced ZMC fractures, the degree of displacement dictates the amount of fixation needed. Stable fixation can be achieved at one-, two-, or three-point fixation in minimally to moderately displaced fractures, while severely displaced/comminuted fractures require four-point fixation. When the zygomaticomaxillary buttress is plated, malar projection is restored, which its maximum point of projection in the frontal view is 10 mm lateral and 20 mm inferior to the lateral canthus. Axial cuts can be obtained and analyzed intraoperatively to adequately verify anteroposterior malar projection, bone reduction, and contrast it to the unaffected site if there is one. Mirroring technique can be utilized too if further bilateral symmetry is needed.

Reduction of the zygomaticofrontal buttress leads to the reestablishment of the vertical projection of the lateral orbit. Accessing the site is performed based on operator preference. This buttress has a narrow interface and might not be as helpful during reduction of rotated fractures. Intraoperative navigation can help assist with this problem by evaluating the position of the rotated segment and adjusting the plating as needed. In addition, due to its proximity to the ZS suture, there are instances in which further dissection is performed to evaluate the ZS reduction. This is with risks on its own, like damage to nearby structures, bleeding, hematoma formation, and the need to appropriately close any dead space and resuspension of soft tissues. Navigation permits the visualization of the reduction of the ZS without having to dissect the tissues of the internal lateral orbit, leading to less potential complications with the benefit of good analysis of reduction. In addition, reduction of the fractures in this area can also be analyzed intraoperatively. Coronal views can be inspected to verify proper vertical projection and reduction.

In the setting or orbital component of ZMC fractures, reduction of the floor or the orbital rim might be needed. In many other instances, the reduction of the other components of the ZMC fracture leads to an appropriate reduction of the orbital floor component. Navigation can be used to evaluate for orbital floor reduction in cases where ZMC has been reduced at its other components. This prevents the unnecessary opening of the orbit, and all its risks, as well as leading to intraoperative evaluation of the reduction of the floor. On the other hand, navigation can also give appropriate information in case of those fractures not being adequately reduced, necessitating operative intervention for further repair. As it will be described in another section, orbital floor reconstruction can be evaluated too for proper volume restoration.

Navigation also facilitates proper reconstruction in complex cases like comminuted fractures, bone defects, delayed surgery, resections, and in cases where landmarks are lost. Navigation software provides a template for correction of butrresess for final functional and cosmetic result as described. In the case of comminution and bone defects, three-dimensional positioning is hard to accomplish as reference points and key landmarks might be lost. Intraoperative evaluation after plating every buttress guide surgery, but with navigation, this can be evaluated in a three-dimensional plane. This can help adjust plates and screws to obtain the desired contours, adjust grafting materials for the same purpose. As mentioned before, in the case of delayed treatment of ZMC fractures, Gong et al. demonstrated good outcomes when using navigation where bilateral differences less than 2 mm was noted in 71.8% of the navigation group while only 35.9% in the traditional non-navigation group.

3 Application of Navigation in Orbital Trauma

Trauma to the orbit commonly causes an increase in its volume, leading to soft tissue herniation and changes of position of its contents. This is due to the structural weakness of floor and medial wall fractures, which is why most of the fractures in the orbit happen in those regions. This can lead to entrapment, diplopia, enophthalmos, and hypoglobus. It is imperative that these fractures are repaired as they can lead to functional and cosmetic issues, and many times secondary surgery is needed.

Fractures of the orbit can be linear, blow out or blow in. Generally, linear fracture patterns retain their periosteal attachments, minimizing the herniation of soft tissues into adjacent structures. Blow out is the most common, being the anterior medial wall, followed by the medial wall, and then the roof, in order of decreasing frequency, the most involved. Blow in fractures are more common in pediatric patients due to the resiliency and flexibility of their bones. These are emergencies as they entrap the muscles, leading to ischemia.

Limited visibility is one of the main contributors to the inability to verify implant position during surgery. This can lead to suboptimal placement of the implant, resulting in unsatisfactory outcomes requiring a secondary surgery. Intraoperative navigation can function to minimize that limited visibility and aid in the proper placement of the desired implant, as well as to verify that the proper dimensions are also being established.

In previous studies, Zavattero et al. found that volume analysis of reconstructed orbits using navigation as compared to reconstructed orbits without navigation yielded a closer result to the unaffected orbit [6]. In addition, they found that there was increase in globe projection in the navigation group potentially due to the higher reliability of reconstruction of the medial wall and orbital floor fractures. Diplopia was also noted to be lower in the navigation group, and none of the navigation group patient required re-exploration and manipulation of the implant, while in the traditional non-navigation group, 20% of the subject did require reoperation.

Surgical planning usually begins with scanning the unaffected orbit and using the mirroring feature onto the affected site. This can be frequently combined with custom-made implants targeted to establish the normal anatomy and volume in these complex cases [7], but stock plates can also be used. With navigation, titanium mesh can be contoured and positioned at the precise location to restore volume and shape of the orbit [8]. Some of the advantages of navigation include immediate feedback during dissection of tissues, removal of bony shattered fragments, spatial awareness leading to the localization of vital structures and adjustments needed throughout the placement of the implant. Among those structures, the anterior and posterior ethmoidal arteries are encountered, which are in general 24 mm and 36 mm posterior to the anterior lacrimal crest in the medial wall of the orbit. In addition, the optic canal is 6 mm posterior to the posterior ethmoidal foramina. Navigation allows for the visualization of the optic canal area when seating the implant or during cauterization of the posterior ethmoidal artery. Position of instruments and the implant can be obtained in real time by having those being probed by the pointer. Those can then be adjusted to match a virtual template if one was created.

The correct reconstruction of the floor of the orbit with the appropriate anatomical contours is paramount for restoring adequate volume. These surgeries can become even more difficult when there is not a posterior ledge for a plate to rest on or when key landmarks are lost. This makes the re-establishment of the orbital volume very challenging as one must consider the vital structures in the orbital apex as well as the musculature in the enclosed space. In orbital wall and medial wall fractures, the extent of the fracture can be analyzed with navigation during their exposure. Once the fractures have been exposed, plates can be placed in position and analyzed in real time before fixation. In addition, herniated tissues can be identified in real time, so that the proper reduction of those is performed before fixation as well as verification of their proximity to the optic canal, minimizing the risk of injuries to the vital structures encountered in that area. Also, this can help minimize the amount of dissection needed for proper exposure in cases where visualization is hard. On the other hand, there are times where adjustments are needed to the plate or the dissection obtained, leading to resistance of passive implant seating. Navigation can allow the surgeon to better identify the area that is interfering with passive implant placement or perform contour changes to the implant based on the working anatomy of the patient and the projections needed. Also, once the implant is fixated, navigation can provide an analysis of the placement and volumetric contours of the orbit, globe, and extraocular muscle position (Fig. 3).

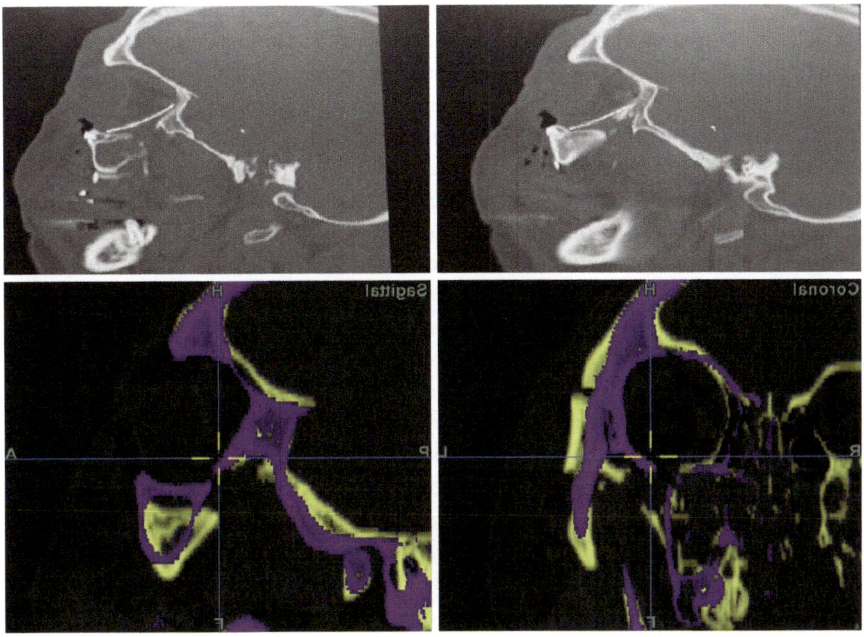

Fig. 3 Orbit fracture navigation guided reconstruction post-op CT comparison

4 Application of Navigation in Foreign Body Removal

Maxillofacial region is constantly encountered with trauma coming from different type of penetrating injuries. Many times, the offending agent can be retained within the confines of this region. Frequently, the location of such objects can be difficult to assess due to the altered anatomy encountered. The destruction caused by the penetrating object, like in the case of projectiles, is an example of such. In addition, the removal of such objects can also be challenging as those can be found in soft tissue, hard tissue, in close proximity to vital structures and/or access to such areas is very limited or difficult. Also, intraoperatively, searching for the foreign body can be difficult and time consuming especially if we consider that there might be multiple foreign bodies. There have been multiple cases in which intraoperative navigation has been employed to successfully locate those foreign bodies and have them removed in a safely and timely manner. Those bodies can range from projectiles, needles, teeth, among others. The advantages of intraoperative navigation offers reside in the concept of spatial awareness. This technology allows for real-time assessment of the foreign object with a projected distance three-dimensionally from the planned incision site and structures nearby. Considering this, access to retrieve foreign bodies can be done in a less invasive and traumatic way. Less invasive surgery leads to decreased trauma to tissues and faster recovery times.

The proper removal of foreign bodies starts with a good pre-surgical planning. CT scans of the maxillofacial region are usually obtained and used as a template for surgical planning. Once intraoperatively, the navigation systems of choice is used to detect the exact anatomical site where each object resides (Fig. 4). Stein reported the use of navigation in the retrieval of needles in a minimally invasive way [9]. Here, navigation was used to map the needle three-dimensionally and instrumentation was probed in real time. The incision was carefully planned based on the most anterior component of the needle, being careful not to violate any key and vital structures in the process. The incision was a small 1 cm incision. Blunt dissection was performed with the aid of real-time probing. The needle was localized and retrieved in less than 5 min with minimal exploration. Yang et al. [10] reported a navigation-assisted case in which 24 "buckshots" were removed successfully from the left neck and face. In the same manner, Guo et al. [11] reported the use of navigation in the retrieval of third molars into the sublingual, pterygomandibular, and lateral pharyngeal spaces. Sato et al. [12] reported the removal of foreign objects into the maxillary sinus. In general terms, navigation with the aid of probing can give real-time data on instruments and foreign bodies. This can help dictate the best approach for retrieval. Once the foreign body and the anatomical key structures are noted, the planned incision is performed, or the existing injury is utilized. Dissection is then performed, and probing of the instrumentation is then used to have three-dimensional orientation and spatial awareness. Once the object is found, instrumentation can be performed in a safe manner using real-time data that can confirm location of nearby structures in relation to the foreign object. Also, navigation can

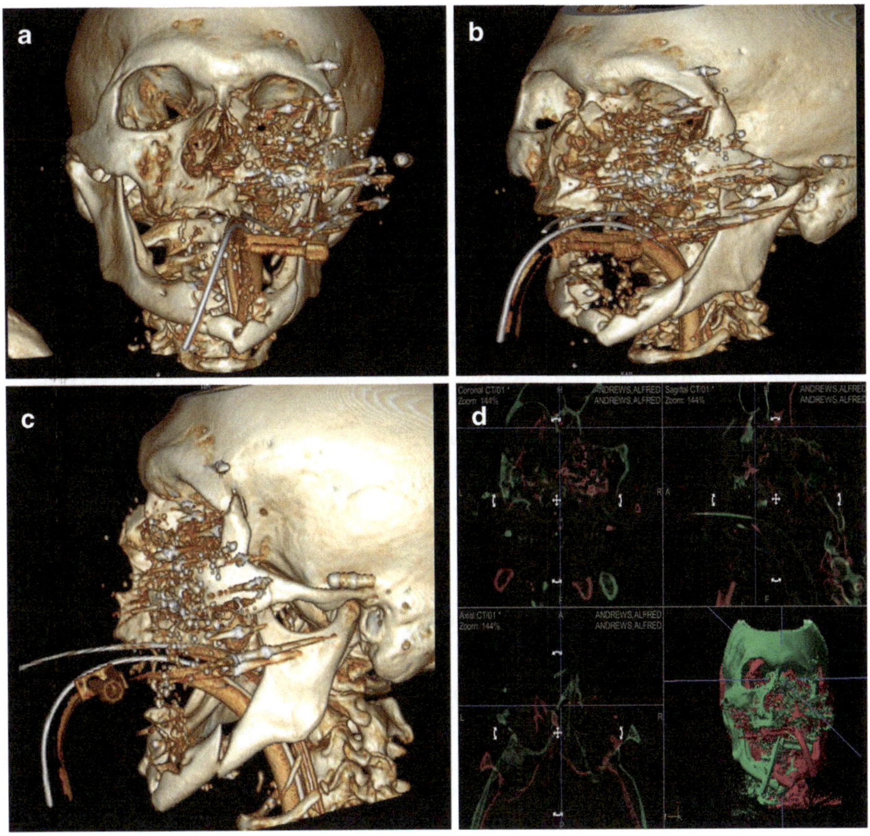

Fig. 4 Identification of fragments/foreign body and assessing contours of reconstruction. (**a**, **b**, **c**) Maxillofacial CT 3D reconstruction of facial gunshot injury. (**d**) Navigation based image correlation of penetrating object location relative to patient anatomy

be used as a tool to confirm all objects have been retrieved when multiple ones as being retrieved.

Time and time again, navigation has proved its value in the retrieval of foreign objects throughout the head and neck region, decreasing incision length, increasing accuracy and time of detection of foreign objects and to verify if those have been removed in case of multiple ones being removed.

5 Limitations of Navigation

Many of the operative management discussed so far has mentioned the use of the mirror feature to aid in proper anatomical repair of the affected side. The use of navigation can be affected in cases where there is bilateral complex trauma, and mirroring is not possible due to the loss of the necessary anatomical landmarks. Furthermore, the use of navigation required the fixation of the reference frame, which can be invasive. This can lead to scarring, infection, injury, and undesirable cosmesis.

One of the main limitations of navigation is the limited use in dynamic systems. Navigation can be successfully used in the midface due to its inherent static position, as compared to a more dynamic mandible. A reference frame is obtained based on the premise that the system is not in constant change. Once change has happened, the accuracy of the reference frame is decreased.

Also, soft tissue changes from the preoperative period to the intraoperative period cannot be effectively corrected. The change in the topographic landmarks of soft tissue leads to a change in the data that was already fixed preoperatively, leading to structural image drift.

Finally, navigation requires extra training for operators and extra cost for patients and many times increased procedure times [13]. There is a steep learning curve, especially in operators that are least experiences in similar equipment.

6 Future of Navigation Surgery

There are different aspects of navigation surgery that are being enhanced for better results intraoperatively. One of those is the ultrasound-guided navigation system which will use ultrasound-based imaging to register the points intraoperatively rather than having this step done preoperatively with CT imaging. This will allow for the correction of soft tissue changes from preop to periop period. Another advancement documented is that of augmented reality-based system. This system incorporates the use of a tracker in the surgeon's headset which allows surgeons to visualize the procedure without the need of moving the head away from the surgical field. In the process, virtual images are converted to real images to allow for better characterization of the operative field [13].

7 Conclusion

Navigation surgery has provided with many advantages to the maxillofacial surgeon in terms of analysis and reconstruction of traumatic injuries to the area. Navigation has been utilized multiple times with satisfactory results ranging from removal of foreign objects, corrects re-approximation of bone fractures, restoration of adequate dimensions, 3D spatial awareness, and assessment of the proximity of vital structures. The current uses provide a framework to keep building on for more complex surgeries and to keep innovating for more advanced systems to correct for the limitations encountered.

References

1. Bell RB. Computer planning and intraoperative navigation in Cranio-maxillofacial surgery. Oral Maxillofac Surg Clin North Am. 2010;22(1):135–56.
2. Dubois L, Schreurs R, Jansen J, Maal T, Essig H, Gooris P, Becking A. Predictability in orbital reconstruction: a human cadaver study. Part II: navigation-assisted orbital reconstruction. J Craniomaxillofac Surg. 2015;43(10):2042–9.
3. Gong X, He Y, An J, Yang Y, Huang X, Liu M, et al. Application of a computer-assisted navigation system (CANS) in the delayed treatment of zygomatic fractures: a randomized controlled trial. J Oral Maxillofac Surg. 2016;75(7):1450–63.
4. Zhang X, Ye L, Li H, Wang Y, Dilxat D, Liu W, et al. Surgical navigation improves reductions accuracy of unilateral complicated zygomaticomaxillary complex fractures: a randomized controlled trial. Sci Rep. 2018;8(1):6890–9.
5. Ogino A, Onishi K, Maruyama Y. Intraoperative repositioning assessment using navigation system in zygomatic fracture. J Craniofac Surg. 2009;20:1061–5. https://doi.org/10.1097/SCS.0b013e3181abb2e8.
6. Zavattero E, Ramieri G, Roccia F, Gerbino G. Comparison of the outcomes of complex orbital fracture repair with and without a surgical navigation system: a prospective cohort study with historical controls. Plastic Reconstr Surg. 2017;139:957–65. https://doi.org/10.1097/PRS.0000000000003229.
7. Feng F, et al. Mirror imaging and preshaped titanium plates in the treatment of unilateral malar and zygomatic arch fractures. Oral Surg Oral Med Oral Pathol Oral Radiol Endod. 2011;112:188–94. https://doi.org/10.1016/j.tripleo.2010.10.014.
8. Yu H, Shen G, Wang X, Zhang S. Navigation-guided reduction and orbital floor reconstruction in the treatment of zygomatic-orbital-maxillary complex fractures. J Oral Maxillofac Surg. 2010;68(1):28–34.
9. Stein KM. Use of intraoperative navigation for minimally invasive retrieval of a broken dental needle. J Oral Maxillofac Surg. 2015;73:1911–6.
10. Yang C, Yang R, He S, Li Z. Removal of a large number of foreign bodies in the maxillofacial region with navigation system. Dent Traumatol. 2017;33(3):230–4. https://doi.org/10.1111/edt.12313.
11. Guo Y, Xu DD, Lv K, Wan QL, Li ZB, Li Z. Use of computer-assisted navigation in the retrieval of accidentally displaced third molars. J Oral Maxillofac Surg. 2016;74:889–94.
12. Sato H, Shiogama S, Narihira K, Chikuda J, Nakamura S, Abe Y, et al. Removal of small foreign bodies from the maxillary sinus using CT image-guided surgical navigation and rapid paired-point registration and calibration with reference markers on an occlusal splint. Oral Maxillofac Surg Cases. 2018;5(1):100089.
13. Anand M, Panwar S. Role of navigation in oral and maxillofacial surgery: a surgeon's perspectives. Clin Cosmet Investig Dent. 2021;13:127–39.

Surgical Navigation in Oral and Maxillofacial Pathology

Waleed Zaid, Andrew Yampolsky, and Beomjune Kim

1 Introduction

The head and neck region is one of the most anatomically and functionally complex structures in the body. In addition, it harbors many critical organs including the brain, eyes, ears, upper airway, pharynx, cranial nerves, and blood vessels. Thus, any pathology arising in this area is particularly challenging to manage surgically. Many technological advances were achieved over the last three decades to overcome the anatomic and functional complexity of head and neck region. These include Digital Imaging and Communications in Medicine (DICOM), Computer-Aided Design and Manufacturing (CAD/CAM), image-guided surgery (IGS)/surgical navigation, and advanced imaging modalities such as intraoperative computed tomography [1] and positron emission tomography (PET). These technologies made possible preoperative surgical simulation and planning with three dimensional images or models, intraoperative image-guided surgery, custom fabricated surgical guides for precise resection and reconstruction, and real-time verification of surgical accuracy.

W. Zaid
Department of Oral and Maxillofacial Surgery, Louisiana State University Health Sciences Center—School of Dentistry, New Orleans, LA, USA
e-mail: Wzaid@lsuhsc.edu

A. Yampolsky
Department of Oral and Maxillofacial Surgery, Sidney Kimmel Medical College, Thomas Jefferson University Hospital, Philadelphia, PA, USA
e-mail: Andrew.Yampolsky@jefferson.edu

B. Kim (✉)
Department of Head and Neck/Microvascular Reconstructive Surgery, Cancer Treatment Centers of America in Atlanta, Part of City of Hope, Newnan, GA, USA
e-mail: Beomjune.kim@ctca-hope.com

S. A. Parhiz et al. (eds.), *Navigation in Oral and Maxillofacial Surgery*,
https://doi.org/10.1007/978-3-031-06223-0_4

First utilized in neurosurgery, the application of surgical navigation has expanded to skull base surgery and maxillofacial surgery including maxillofacial trauma, dentoalveolar surgery, orthognathic surgery [2], and pathology [3]. In this chapter, we briefly describe several principles behind surgical navigation and discuss the use of surgical navigation in treating head and neck pathology through the presentation of several surgical cases. Surgical navigation allows orientation and positioning of a surgical instrument in a complex three-dimensional anatomic structure. The surgeon can visualize the real-time position of surgical instrument on the computer monitor with the patient-specific imaging data. This technology has greatly improved surgical predictability and accuracy, while minimizing intraoperative invasiveness [4]. The main indications of surgical navigation in head and neck pathology are to ensure adequate tumor margins in areas of difficult visualization, to precisely locate a foreign body [5] or an accidentally displaced tooth [6], to accurately position bony reconstruction or hardware, and to verify the accurate delivery of surgical plan.

2 Principles Behind Image-Guided Surgery (IGS): Surgical Navigation

Image-guided surgery (IGS) has gradually increased in both utilization and capabilities over the past several decades since first becoming commercially available. Within the broad field of head and neck surgery, IGS is most frequently utilized as an adjunctive technique in rhinology and skull base surgery. Increasingly, as experience with IGS has progressed, there have been efforts to utilize IGS for a more diverse set of head and neck surgical applications.

IGS, often referred to as surgical navigation describes systems from several vendors that attempt to provide intraoperative computer-aided anatomical guidance to the surgeon. This is a particular asset in operations that require from limited dissection and exposure, thus making it difficult to identify key anatomical landmarks. Generally, these systems provide an overlay which relates anatomical imaging, often displayed on a screen as coronal, sagittal, and axial sections with a pointer that is meant to relay the position of a pre-registered surgical instrument within the operative field. This is beneficial when operating in an enclosed, poorly visualized space, near vital structures. Given this description, it is not surprising that the American Academy of Otolaryngology currently supports the use of IGS in sinus surgery.

There are several principles that apply to all the intraoperative visualization systems on the market. Anatomic imaging, in the form of either a CT or an MRI must be utilized that accurately represents the anatomy in question. Thus, the imaging must be obtained as close to the planned surgical time frame as possible to ensure minimal changes to the anatomy in question.

The patient anatomy must then be intraoperatively mapped and related to the imaging. This is usually done utilizing fixed fiduciary points which may consist of taped on skin markers, fixed anatomical landmarks such as teeth, or even bone anchored fiduciaries. Other registration techniques include contour-based registration which matches three-dimensional contours traced on the patient with that which is present on the imaging [7]. Additionally, stereotactic frames fixed to the patient intraoperatively may be used. The choice of registration technique depends on the technical demands of the operation being performed [8]. Regardless of the registration technique chosen, it is important to be mindful of registration errors which can be compounded by technical errors during the registration process. Generally, the goal is to have a target registration error of under 2 mm.

3 Case No. 1: Broken Needle

Retrieval of a broken needle from an anatomically complex region can be challenging without surgical navigation. Although this is not a pathology per se, the principles guiding the technique of removing a broken needle can be applied to pathology. The technique has been previously described in multiple articles [5, 9].

This is a case of an 18-year-old African American female patient who was referred with a chief complaint of pain that was started 1 year ago after a general dentist surgically extracted her wisdom teeth. During the administration of inferior alveolar nerve block, a 27-gauge long needle was fractured and trapped in the soft tissue. The dentist was unable to retrieve the needle fragment at the time, and it was decided to leave the needle fragment in its place. The patient was observed for development of symptoms or needle migration.

The patient did not develop any trismus. However, she experienced persistent pain exacerbated during mouth opening and closing. A panoramic radiograph confirmed the needle fragment in the right pterygomandibular space (Fig. 1), and a surgical exploration was recommended.

A preoperative medical grade 1 mm-slice CT scan was taken 1 week prior to surgery to confirm the location of the needle. The DICOM data was uploaded to the Medronic surgical workstation. After the patient was intubated, the electromagnetic field emitter device was mounted to the surgical bed next to the patient's head, while

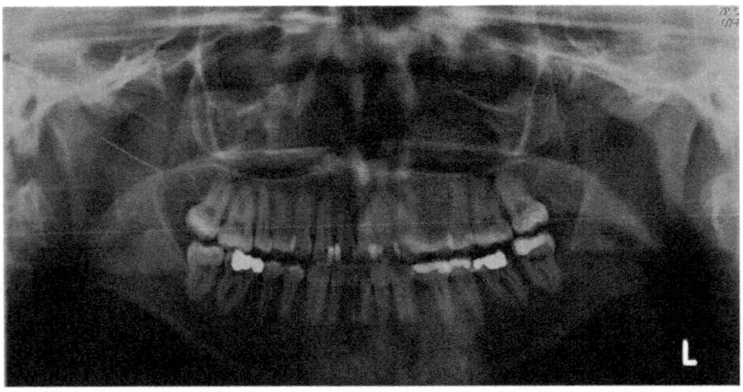

Fig. 1 Panoramic X-ray showing a right broken needle, displaced superior to the inferior alveolar nerve

a tracker device was adhered to the patient's mid-forehead. Patient registration was performed. With a registration probe, a series of points in the forehead, periorbital, and nasal regions were traced. The registration software matched the previously traced points to their corresponding points on the patient's preoperative CT scan. After successful patient registration, movement of the probe instrument corresponded to the same movement on the preoperative CT scan, which was displayed on the workstation monitor. We then verified the accuracy of the patient registration by pointing the tip of the registration probe at various anatomic landmarks, such as the anterior nasal spine, medial canthus, and incisors, ensuring that the software also pointed to the corresponding positions on the preoperative CT scan. The positional discrepancy was verified to be less than 1 mm. The patient was then prepped and draped. The preoperative CT scan indicated that the broken needle was above the lingula and oriented superiorly toward the sigmoid notch. To gain access, a 4 cm vertical incision along the ramus was made. Subperiosteal dissection was carried out medially along the ramus. The lingula and the inferior alveolar nerve were identified. The broken needle could not be visualized or palpated because it was trapped within the medial pterygoid musculature. Next, we positioned the navigation probe until the tip of the instrument was at the most anterior point of the needle fragment on the preoperative CT scan (Fig. 2).

With the navigation probe still in position, blunt dissection was performed adjacent to the probe instrument. The tip of the needle fragment was identified, and the broken needle was retrieved with a hemostat (Fig. 3). Care was taken to ensure that the inferior alveolar nerve was protected during the dissection. No vital structures

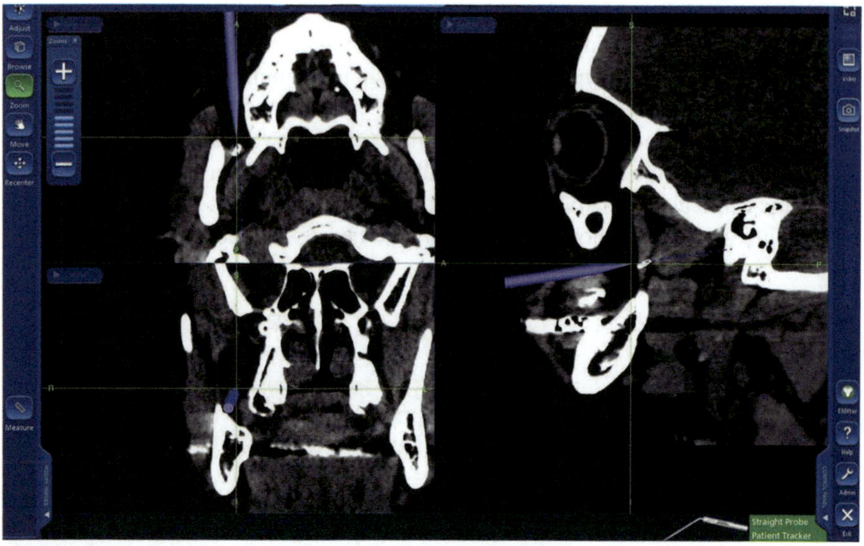

Fig. 2 A screenshot of the navigation monitor showing the navigation probe in relation to the broken needle in the axial, coronal, and sagittal views

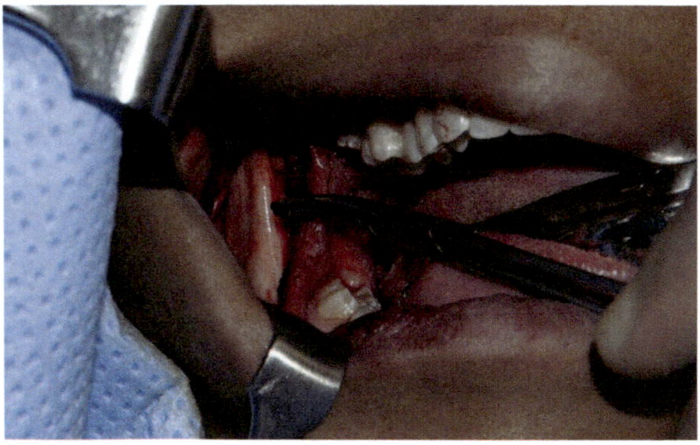

Fig. 3 Intraoperative picture showing the utilization of the mandibular vestibular incision and the retrieval of the broken needle with a hemostat

were injured. The incision was closed with 3-0 chromic sutures. Total intraoperative time was less than 30 min. The patient was discharged home on the same day, and there were no postoperative complications.

4 Case No. 2: Displaced Tooth into the Infratemporal Fossa

This is a case of a 14-year-old male patient, who was referred after a failed attempt of maxillary wisdom tooth extraction. During the extraction attempt, the surgeon did not visualize the tooth completely, and blind elevation was attempted, but the patient moved during the dental elevation, and the operating surgeon could not identify or visualize the tooth anymore. The surgeon decided to abort the procedure and refer the patient for further management.

A medical grade 1 mm-slice CT scan was taken and confirmed a non-completely formed maxillary tooth displaced into the infratemporal fossa. The DICOM data was uploaded to the Medronic surgical workstation. After the patient was intubated, the electromagnetic field emitter device was mounted to the surgical bed next to the patient's head, a tracker device was adhered to the patient's mid-forehead. Patient registration was performed. We used a tracer registration probe to trace a series of points in the forehead, periorbital, and nasal regions. The registration software matched the previously outlined points to their corresponding points on the patient's preoperative CT scan (Fig. 4). After successful patient registration, movement of the probe instrument corresponded to the same movement on the preoperative CT scan, which was displayed on the workstation monitor. We then verified the accuracy of the patient registration by pointing the tip of the registration probe at various anatomic landmarks, such as the anterior nasal spine, medial canthus, and incisors, ensuring that the software also pointed to the corresponding positions on the preoperative CT scan (Fig.5). A classic vestibular incision was used to expose the posterior maxilla. This is a conservative approach to the infratemporal fossa as opposed to a more invasive hemi-coronal approach, along with the lip split ± mandibulotomy utilized for oncologic resection (Fig.6).

Using a navigation suction tip was used to constantly verify the position of the displaced wisdom tooth on the navigation monitor. Blunt dissection was carried out

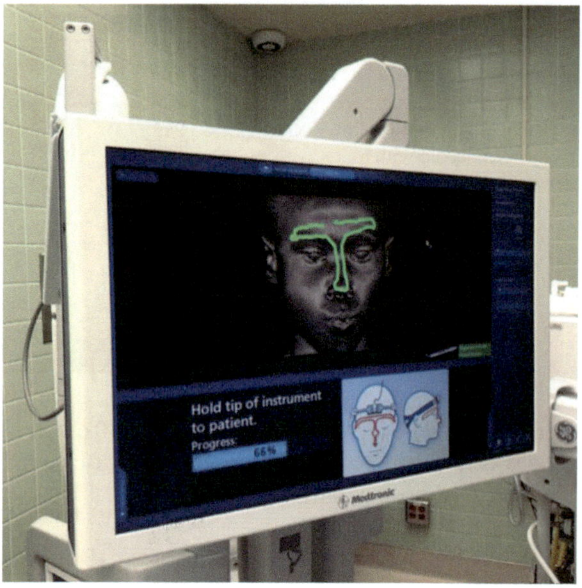

Fig. 4 Tracer registration probe used to trace out a series of points in the forehead, periorbital, and nasal regions

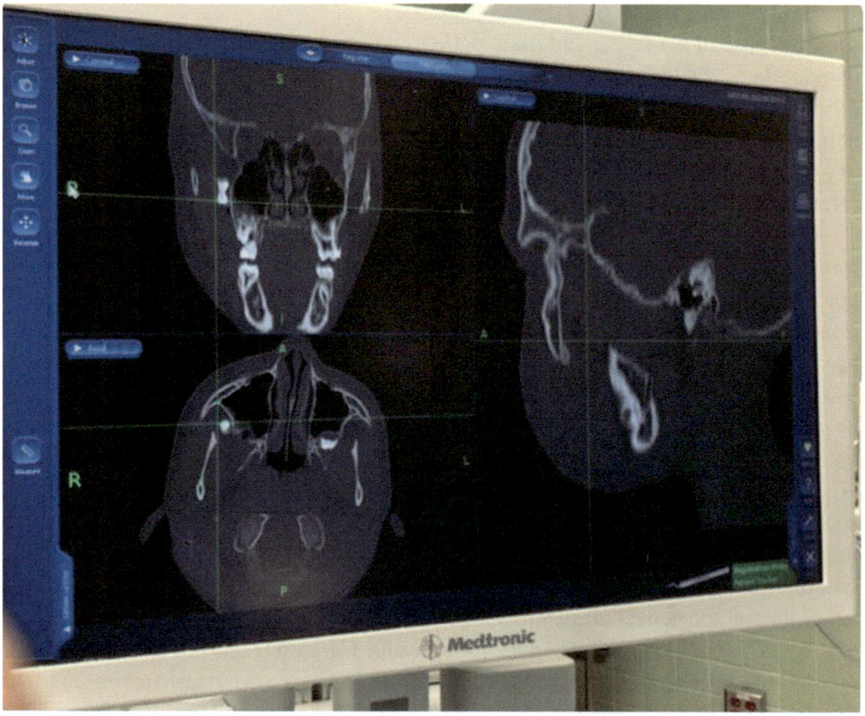

Fig. 5 Accuracy of the registration is confirmed, and locating the displaced maxillary third molar tooth was done in the axial, coronal, and sagittal views

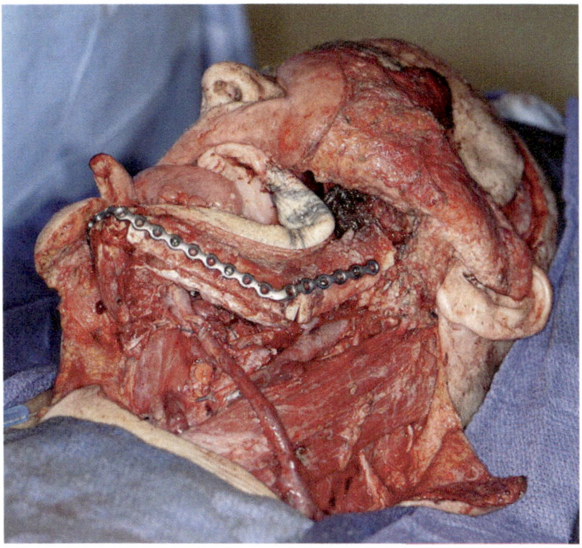

Fig. 6 A case of oral squamous cell carcinoma with infratemporal fossa extension approached with a lip split mandibulectomy along with the hemicoronal approach. Note in this case the mandible was resected and a free vascularized fibula free flap was used as a reconstruction modality

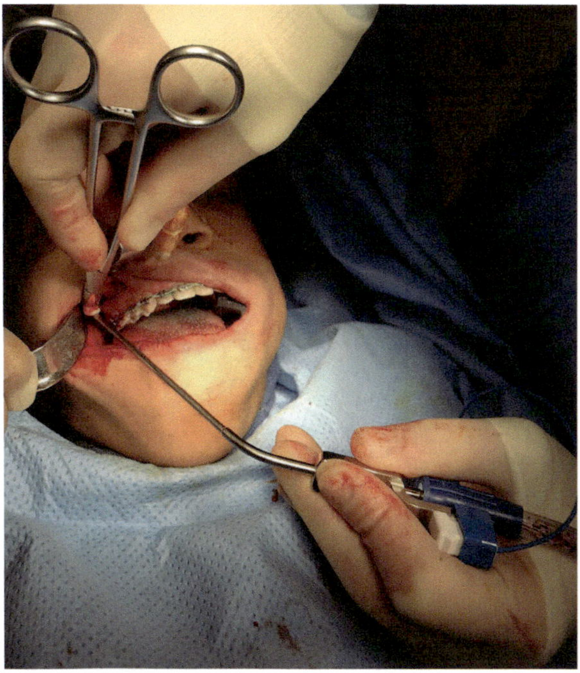

Fig. 7 The tooth was grabbed with a hemostat and retrieved via a transoral vestibular maxillary incision; note the navigation suction tip

until the tooth was palpated with the suction tip where a fibrous capsule was started to form around it. This was incised using electrocautery, and the tooth was retrieved with a hemostat (Fig. 7). The vestibular incision was closed in the standard fashion. A displaced third molar in the maxillary sinus can be located and retrieved using the same technique [10].

5 Case No. 3: Maxillary Tumor/Ossifying Fibroma

This is a case of a 35-year-old female, mentally challenged non-verbal syndromic patient, who was trach dependent, PEG tube dependent, and bed-ridden. Her past medical history is significant for cerebral palsy, hydrocephalus treated with a ventriculoperitoneal shunt, hyperparathyroidism, epilepsy, and asthma (Fig. 8). She was referred for purulent drainage from the left eye and was treated with antibiotics. A clinical exam was not possible. However, a maxillofacial CT scan showed a left maxillary mass, eroding into the orbital space superiorly, nasal cavity medially, the palate inferiorly and posteriorly into the pterygoid plates. The mass had eroded into the left orbital floor and medial orbital wall and was very close to the optic canal (Fig. 9).

An outside biopsy from the referring doctor suggested that this mass is a fibro-osseous lesion that is consistent with fibrous dysplasia; however, this did not correlate with our clinical and radiographic findings. Because of her complex medical history, we recommended excisional biopsy in the form of a hemi-maxillectomy with patient-specific custom plates to reconstruct the midface. The resection was planned through a transfacial approach utilizing a modified Weber-Ferguson

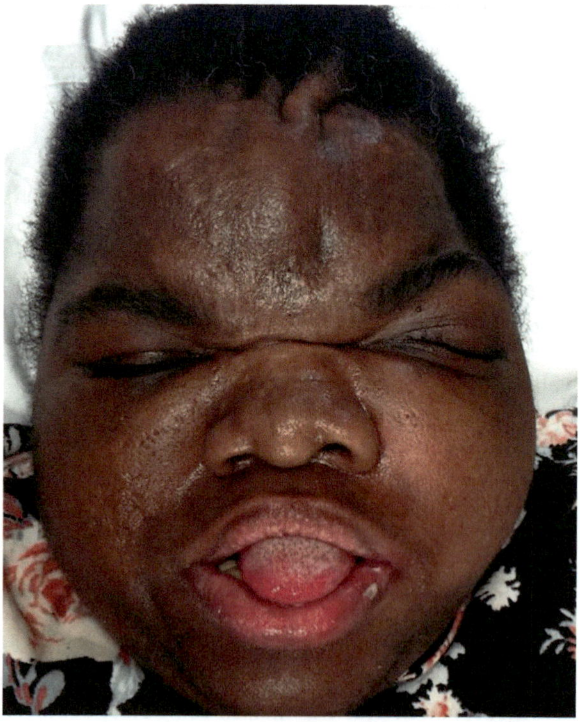

Fig. 8 Frontal view of the patient, showing slight facial swelling on the L side of the midface

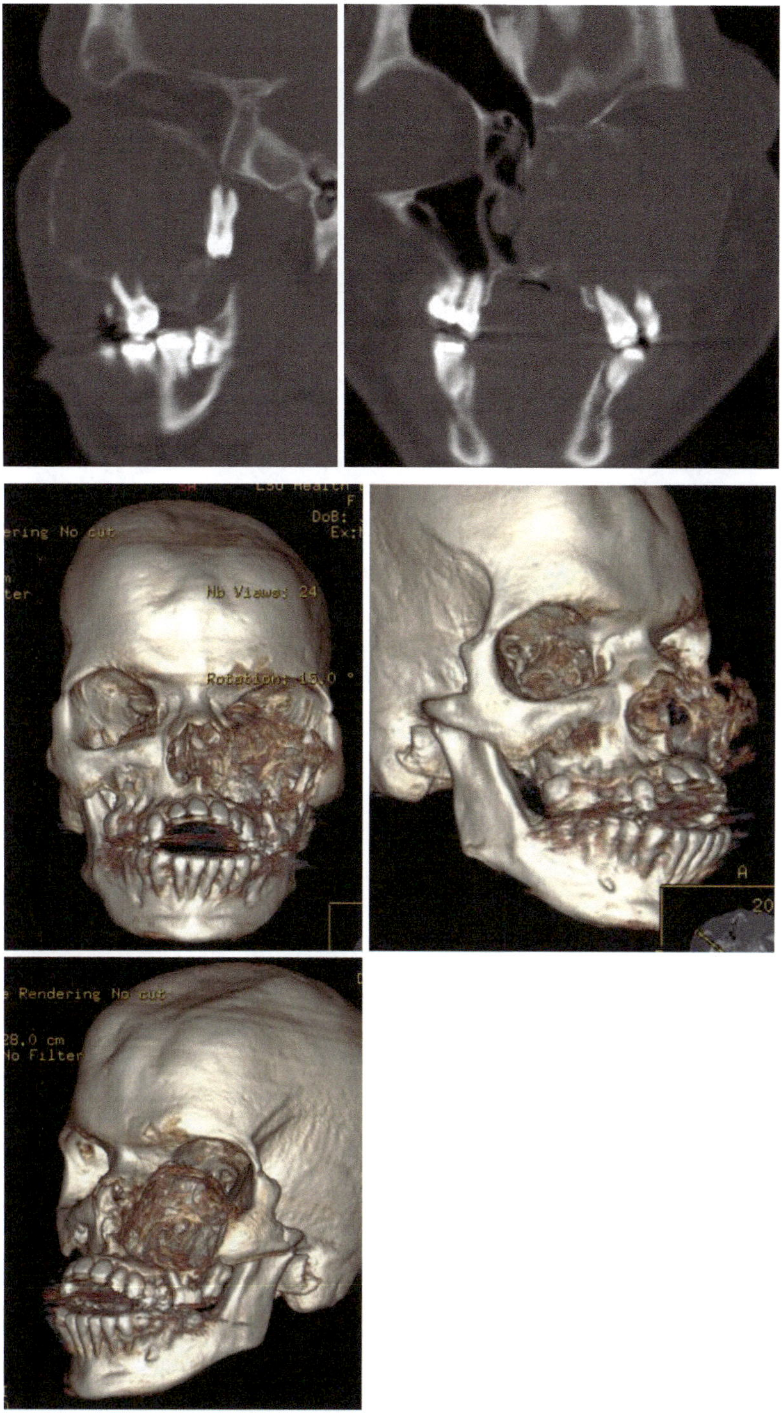

Fig. 9 Selected cuts from the CT scan showing L maxillary mass eroding into the L orbital floor, L medial orbital wall, L palatal bone, and nasal cavity

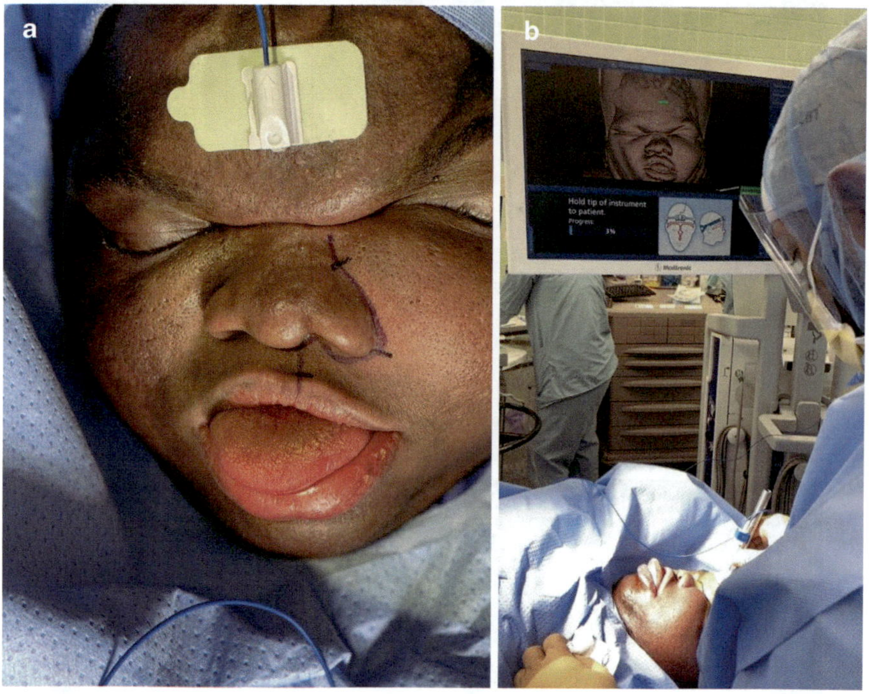

Fig. 10 (**a**) Modified Weber-Ferguson approach outline for a transfacial approach. (**b**) Patient registration with tracing probe

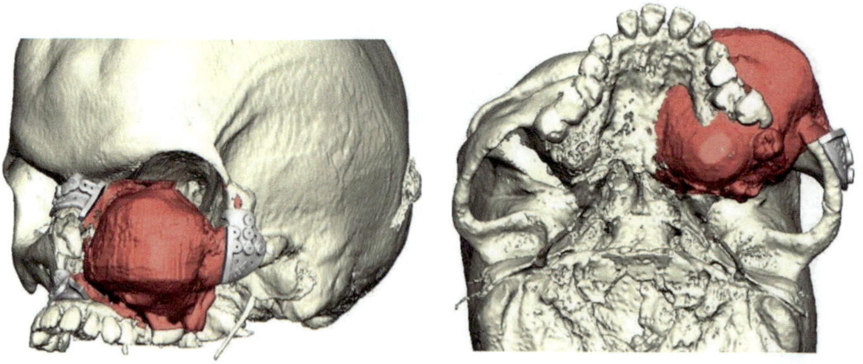

Fig. 11 Planned resection of the maxillary mass, utilizing cutting guides, while the posterior resection margin was aided with navigation

approach (Fig. 10). The Medronic navigation was used similarly to the previous two cases to verify the posterior resection margin, verify safe distance from the optic canal and the globe (Fig. 11). The rest of the resection was aided with surgical cutting guides to assure surgical clearance of the mass.

Intraoperatively, the mass did not have an infiltrative behavior and was easily dissected with clear anatomic planes between the mass and the adjacent tissues (Fig. 12). The superior dissection revealed no invasion into the periorbital fat. After the mass was completely excised, the custom midface plate was secured in place to recreate the medial and inferior orbital walls (Figs. 13 and 14). Final pathology result was reported as ossifying fibroma.

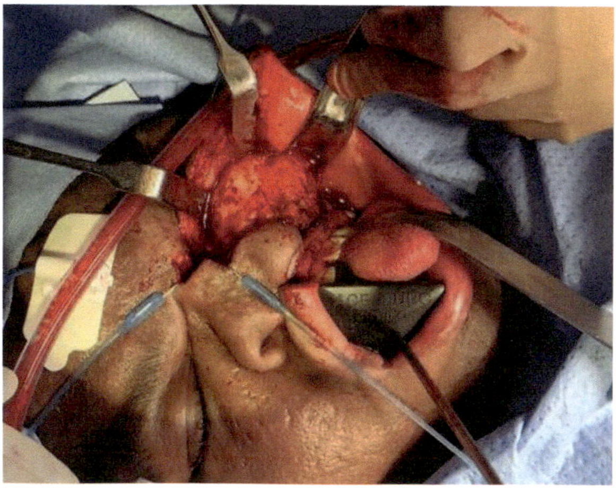

Fig. 12 Exposure of the maxillary mass

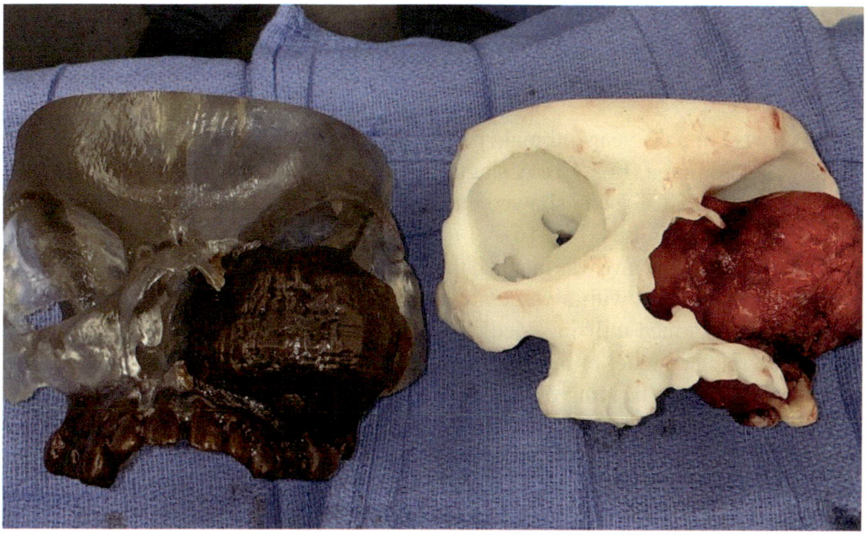

Fig. 13 The maxillary mass was resected and compared with the preoperative surgical model

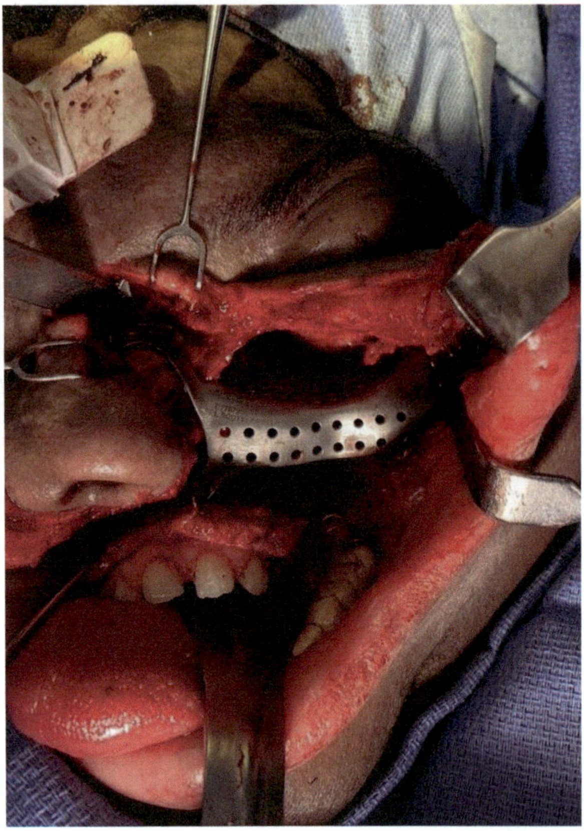

Fig. 14 Custom-made midface plate fixated to the nasal bone, native anterior maxilla, and the body of the zygoma laterally

6 Case No. 4: Maxillary Squamous Cell Carcinoma

This is a case of a 63-year-old male patient presenting with stage 4 maxillary squamous cell carcinoma (Fig. 15). A staging positron emission tomography/computed tomography (PET-CT) scan showed extensive tumor involvement of the nasal cavity and maxillary sinuses (Fig. 16).

Subtotal maxillectomy was planned through a transoral approach. Maxillary reconstruction was planned with a vascularized fibula free flap. Virtual surgical planning (VSP) was performed utilizing Medical Modeling Software (Fig. 17). In addition, a stereolithographic model of the reconstructed maxilla was fabricated for a visual aid and template for pre-bending the plates (Fig. 18). A modified DICOM was generated by superimposing the virtually planned fibula images to the DICOM data of patient's preoperative CT (Fig. 19). This was imported into the navigation workstation.

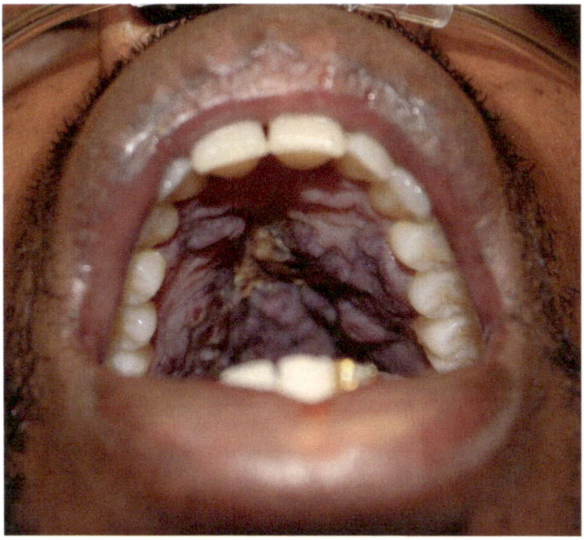

Fig. 15 Extensive involvement of the maxilla by squamous cell carcinoma

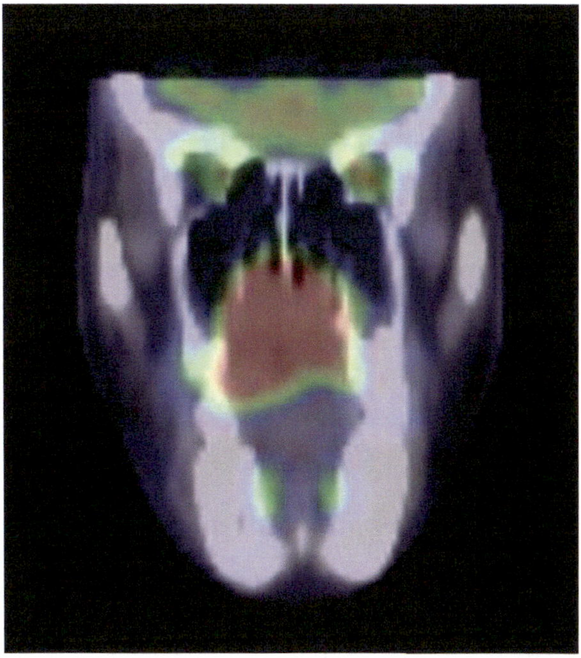

Fig. 16 A PET-CT revealing extensive involvement of the nasal cavity and maxillary sinuses by the tumor

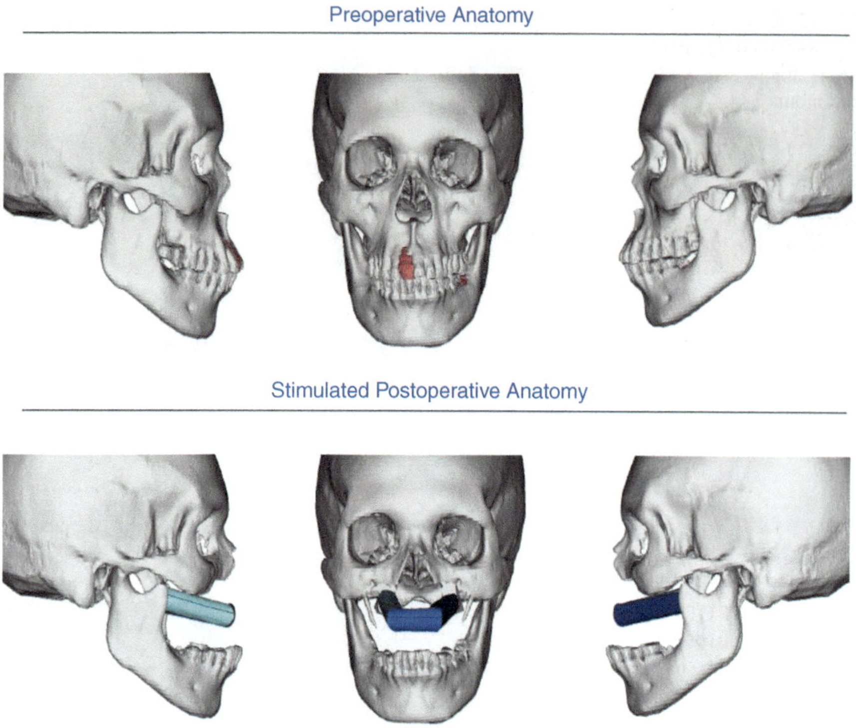

Fig. 17 Virtual surgical plan (VSP) showing the resected and reconstructed maxilla with fibula free flap

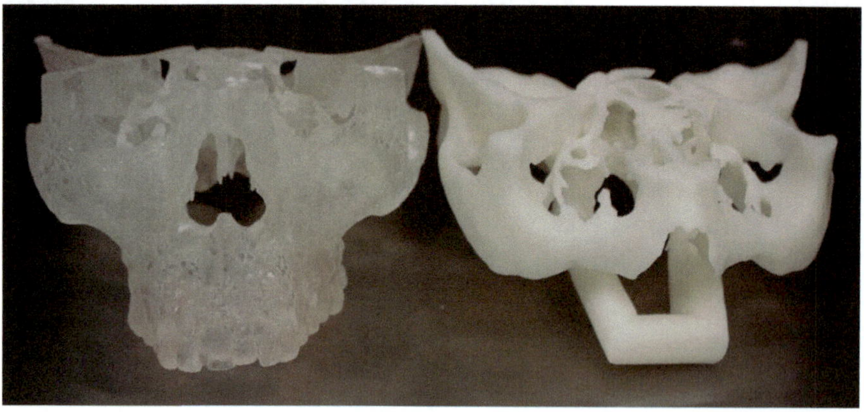

Fig. 18 Stereolithographic model of the reconstructed maxilla

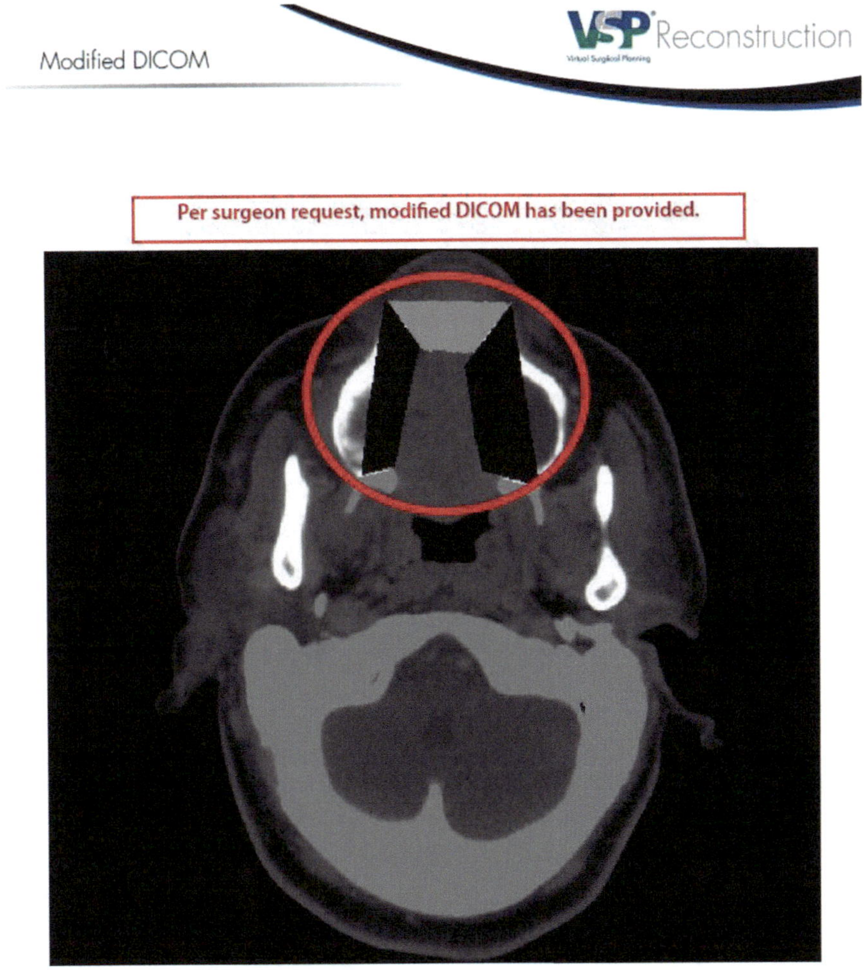

Fig. 19 A modified DICOM combining the virtually planned fibula and DICOM data of patient's preoperative CT

Intraoperatively, the Stryker Navigation System was used to verify the superior resection margin and verify the safe distance from the skull base (Fig. 20). With the use of surgical navigation, the exact position of the tip of any surgical instrument can be evaluated as the instrument is being used, including the tip of the reciprocating saw in this case during septal osteotomy near the skull base.

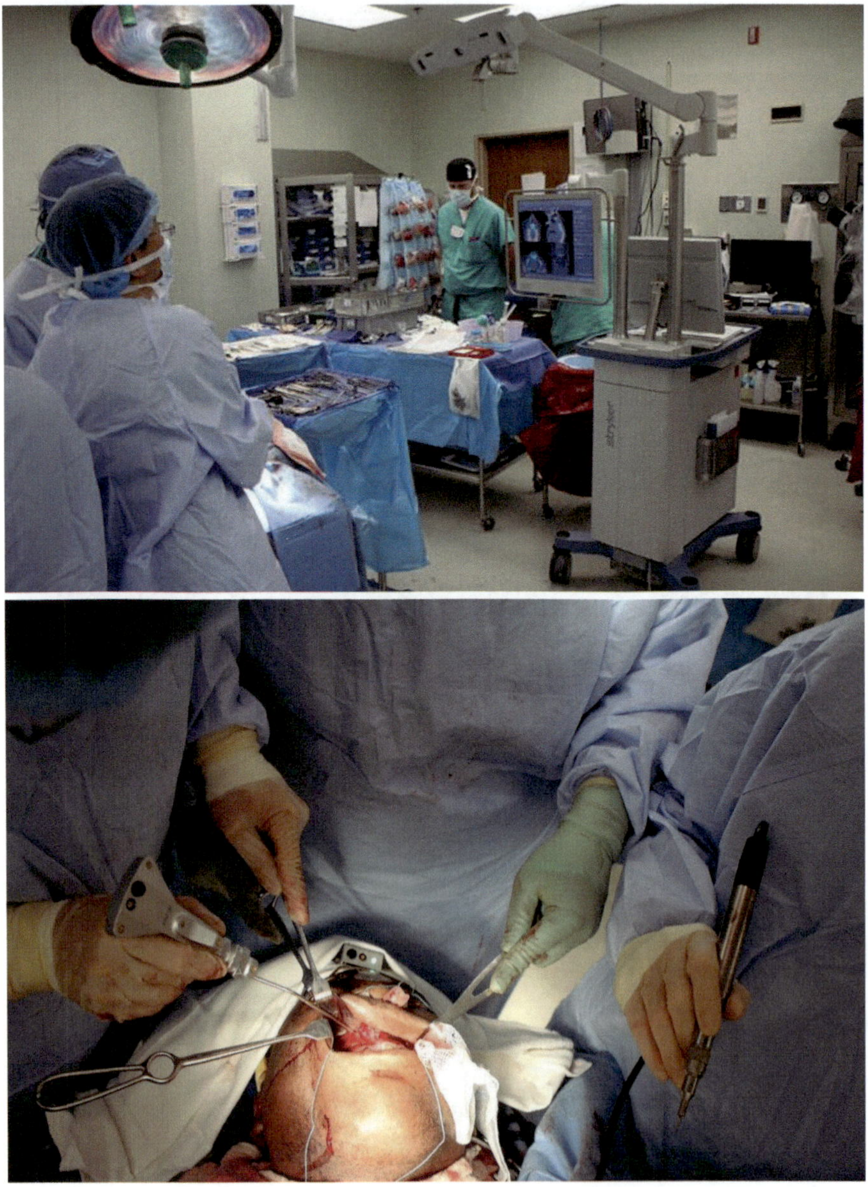

Fig. 20 Verification of the resection margins with surgical navigation

Transoral positioning of the fibula flap in a total or sub-total maxillary defect is an extremely challenging task due to the limited visibility in the posterior maxillary defect, especially when the pterygoid plates have been removed. In this case, a modified DICOM data provided reference points for verification of the fibula position (Fig. 21). After the adequate positioning of the fibula segments was verified by navigation, the neo-maxilla was secured to the zygoma and nasal bone with multiple mid-face plates (Fig. 22). A postoperative CT confirmed an accurate reproduction of the preplanned reconstruction (Fig. 23).

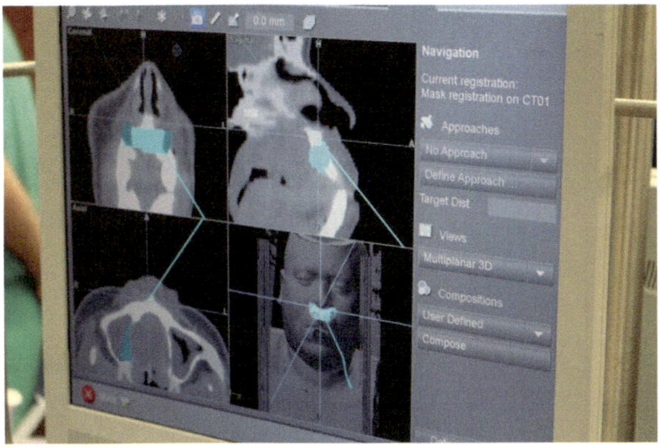

Fig. 21 Verification of the fibula flap using surgical navigation

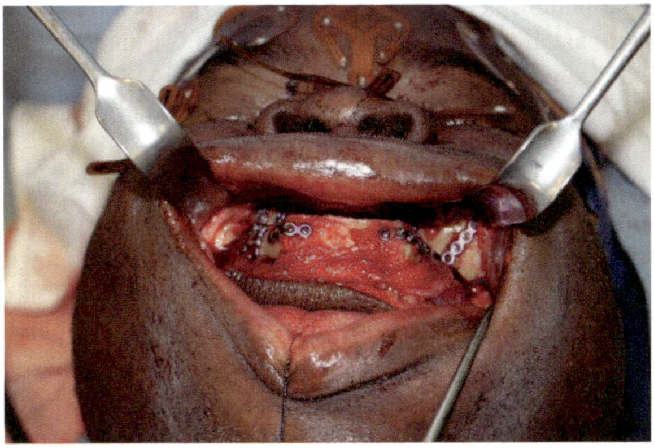

Fig. 22 Reconstructed maxilla with fibula

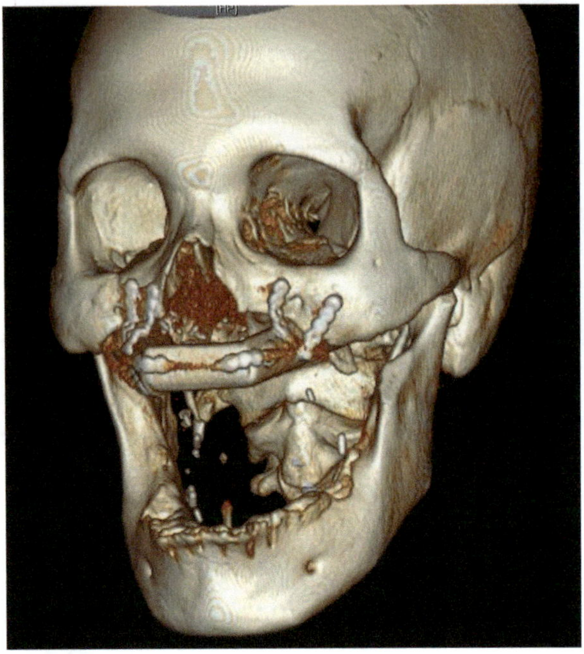

Fig. 23 Postoperative CT showing an adequate position of the reconstructed maxilla

7 Case No. 5: Infratemporal Fossa Tumor

The patient is a 47-year-old woman referred for evaluation of a rapidly enlarging left palatal mass. Work-up consisted of CT and MRI followed by an incisional transoral biopsy which revealed the diagnosis of cT4aN0 adenoid cystic carcinoma of the right maxillary sinus. Imaging suggested that there was no evidence of orbital involvement (Fig. 24). However, the mass did involve the infratemporal fossa, and there was evidence of widening of the foramen ovale and the mass approached the orbital apex. The decision was made to take the patient for a subtotal maxillectomy with orbital preservation, immediate reconstruction with a parascapular free flap. It was also decided that given the likely involvement of the skull base, intraoperative navigation would be utilized to assist with identification of anatomical landmarks and to ensure clearance of this complex anatomical region.

The navigation system utilized in this case was manufactured by Stryker and utilized the Cranial Map 3.0 Software as well as the Cranial Mask Tracker. This is an optical tracking system that measures infrared (IR) light transmitted from the tracked object and requires line of site to function. Given the planned combined transoral and transfacial approach, care was taken to position the Cranial Mask Tracker in a manner where it will not be displaced or distorted by retraction (Fig. 25). In addition, care was also taken to utilize landmarks that would not be distorted or moved by the dissection and retraction process. For instance, the right canthus and nasal tip were not utilized as they would likely result in distortion and target localization errors.

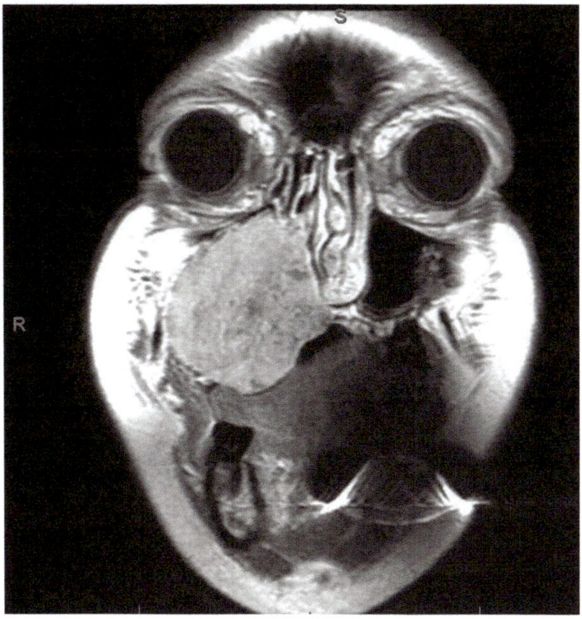

Fig. 24 T1-weighted coronal MRI slice demonstrating the aggressive sino-nasal adenoid cystic carcinoma effacing the right maxillary sinus and approaching the orbit

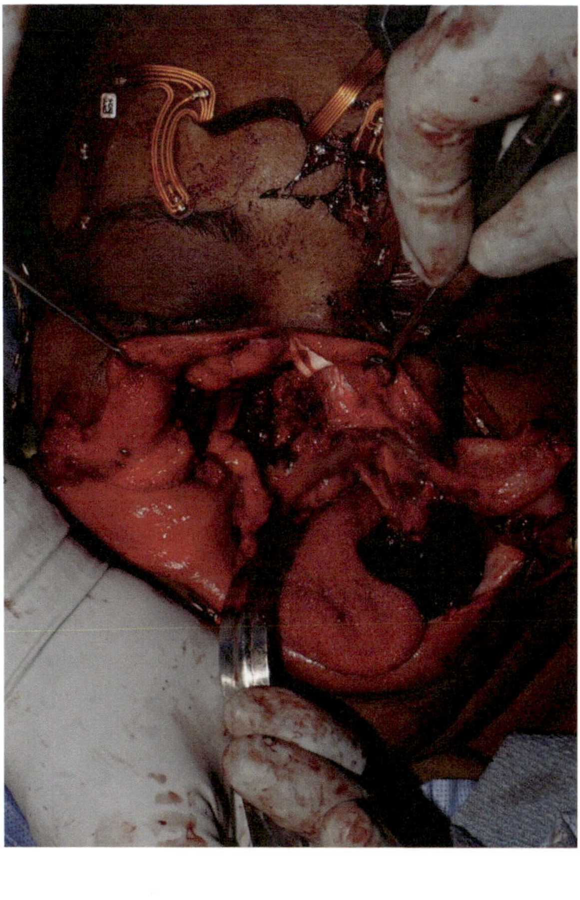

Fig. 25 Intraoperative photograph demonstrating the positioning of the cranial mask tracker and surgical approach. Note the distortion of landmarks by retraction

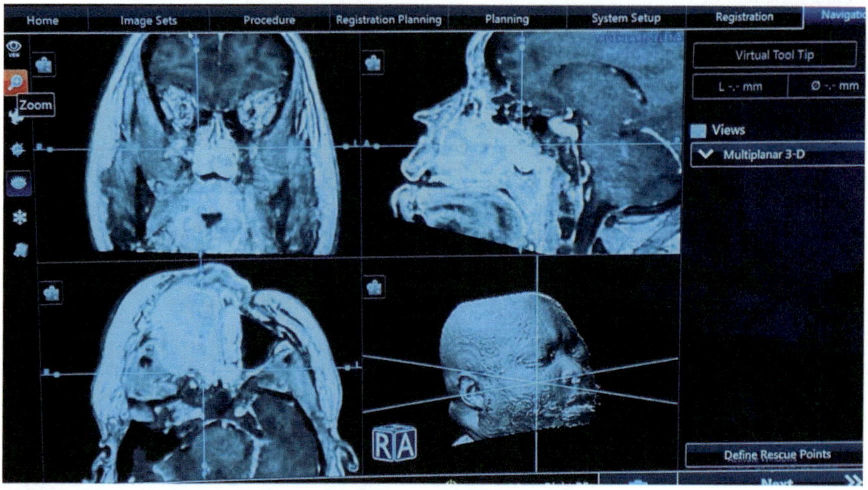

Fig. 26 The anatomical information provided intraoperatively via the Stryker navigation system

A subtotal maxillectomy, including the right orbital floor, but sparing the orbital contents was performed without complication. Navigation was used to help Identify cranial base skeletal landmarks including the pterygoid canal, and foramen ovale (Fig. 26). This helped ensure clearance of all soft tissue in this region and assisted with tracing the mandibular nerve to the foramen and obtaining adequate specimens of the nerve for intraoperative pathologic consultation.

8 Case No. 6: Mandibular Tumor

A less common application for intraoperative navigation is surgery involving the mandible. Unlike surgery involving the maxilla and cranial base, the mandible is by nature a mobile structure owing to its articulation at the temporomandibular joint [11]. In the following case, we describe a simple method to work around this limitation while still maintaining a high degree of tracking accuracy.

The patient is a 22-year-old woman who has a history of a mandibular ameloblastoma that was managed conservatively with enucleation and curettage by another surgeon 3 years ago. She reports that on a recent radiograph her dentist noticed an unusual radiolucent lesion in her right mandibular ramus. There was concern that this may represent recurrent disease, so the dentist performed an in-office biopsy. This biopsy demonstrated normal trabecular bone which suggested that the area of concern was not adequately sampled.

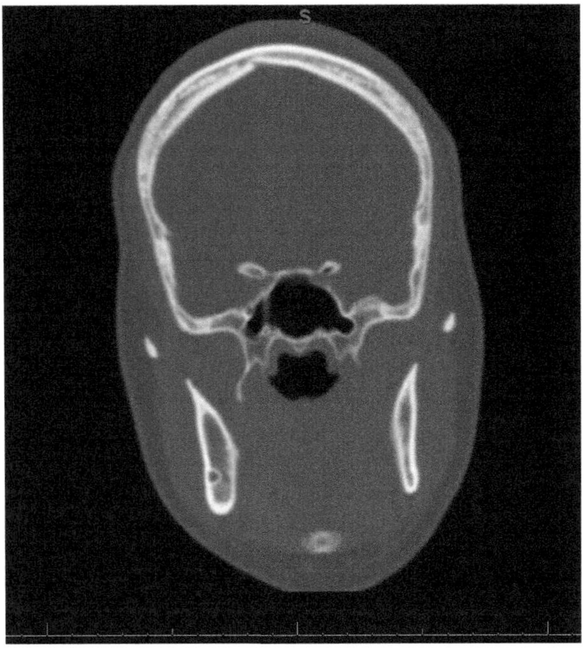

Fig. 27 A coronal cut of a non-contrast-enhanced CT of the facial bones, demonstrating an area in the right mandibular ramus suspicious for recurrent ameloblastoma

As part of evaluation, a CT of the facial skeleton was ordered. When evaluating the CT, we noted several areas of small, less than 5 mm in diameter lytic lesions that had the appearance of a soap bubble (Fig. 27). This was highly suspicious for a recurrence, but given their location, it would be difficult to definitively identify one of these areas for biopsy.

At this point, it was decided that the best course of action would be to perform a biopsy with the aid of stereotactic guidance to definitively identify the area of suspicion while also minimizing morbidity.

The key to utilizing intraoperative navigation in this case was acquiring the reference imaging with the patient in maximum intercuspation [12]. This allowed us to replicate the mandibular position intraoperatively by placing the patient in temporary maxillomandibular fixation. The navigation system utilized in this case was manufactured by Stryker and utilized the Cranial Map 3.0 Software as well as the Cranial Mask Tracker. The dentition was able to be utilized in this case as a very accurate fiduciary marker during registration, in addition to facial landmarks.

A transoral biopsy was performed, utilizing a rotary instrument which was registered and calibrated with the guidance system. This allowed us to make a window osteotomy directly over the area of concern, while minimizing extraneous tissue damage (Fig. 28). The patient tolerated the procedure well, and the biopsy revealed recurrent ameloblastoma. She was subsequently worked up for definitive management.

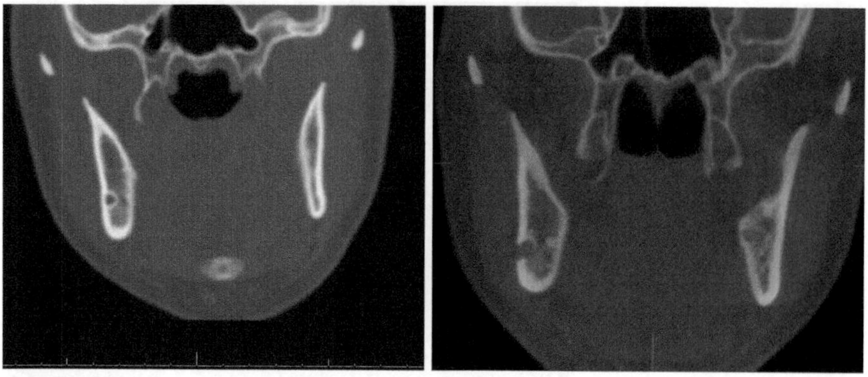

Fig. 28 The accuracy of the corticotomy that provided access to the concerning area

9 Conclusion

As described in this chapter, surgical navigation allows accurate spatial orientation and positioning of anatomic structures. This in turn guides surgeon to locate a relevant anatomic structure even in an invisible area during surgery. Its application in oral and maxillofacial pathology has gradually expanded over the years. It is extremely useful in delineating the location and extent of tumor, locating a foreign body, and accurate positioning of bony segments or reconstruction plates. With the advent of prefabricated cutting/positioning guides with predictive drilling holes and milled/printed reconstruction plates, surgical navigation has less role in positioning of reconstructive bony segments or reconstruction plates. However, it can prove to be helpful when these guides are not available. In addition, it continues to play a significant role in other indications. The technology is continuously evolving to simplify the logistics of operation and to complement other technological modalities. For example, an intraoperative C-arm fluoroscopy or cone-beam CT used in conjunction with surgical navigation can provide real-time anatomic data before and after surgical resection of tumor without having to leave the operating room. In addition, the use of surgical navigation can verify the position of hardware or reconstructed bone after reconstruction was achieved using custom-fabricated reconstruction guides and plates.

References

1. Wm VH, Van Cann EM, Muradin MS, Frank MH, Koole R. Intraoperative imaging for the repair of zygomaticomaxillary complex fractures: a comprehensive review of the literature. J Craniomaxillofac Surg. 2014;42:1918–23.
2. Kang SH, Kim MK, Choi YS, Park W, Lee SH. Navigation assisted intraoral vertical ramus osteotomy. J Oral Maxillofac Surg. 2011;69:931–4.

3. Sukegawa S, Takahiro K, Furuki Y. Application of computer-assisted navigation systems in oral and maxillofacial surgery. Jpn Dent Sci Rev. 2018;54:139–49.
4. Azarmehr I, Stokbro K, Bell RB, Thygesen T. Surgical navigation: a systematic review of indications, treatments, and outcomes in oral and maxillofacial surgery. J Oral Maxillofac Surg. 2017;75:1987–2005.
5. Wei R, Xiang-Zhen L, Bing G, Da-Long S, Ze-Ming. Removal of a foreign body from the skull base using a customized computer-designed guide bar. J Craniomaxillofac Surg. 2010;38:279–83.
6. Campbell A, Costello BJ. Retrieval of a displaced third molar using navigation and active image guidance. J Oral Maxillofac Surg. 2010;68:480–5.
7. Li L, Yang J, Chu Y, Wu W, Xue J, Liang P, et al. A novel augmented reality navigation system for endoscopic sinus and skull base surgery: a feasibility study. PLoS One. 2016;11(1):e0146996.
8. Luebbers HT, Messmer P, Obwegeser JA, Zwahlen RA, Kikinis R, Graetz KW, et al. Comparison of different registration methods for surgical navigation in cranio-maxillofacial surgery. J Craniomaxillofac Surg. 2008;36:109–16.
9. Nezafati S, Shahi S. Removal of broken dental needle using mobile digital C-arm. J Oral Sci. 2008;50:351–3.
10. Iwai T, Matsui Y, Hirota M, Tohnai I. Endoscopic removal of a maxillary third molar displaced into the maxillary sinus via the socket. J Craniofac Surg. 2012;23:e295–6.
11. Casap N, Wexler A, Eliashar R. Computerized navigation for surgery of the lower jaw; comparison of 2 navigation sytems. J Oral Maxillofac Surg. 2008;66:1467–75.
12. Li P, Li Z, Tian W, Tang W. A strategy for removal of foreign body in mandible with navigation system. Int J Oral Maxillofac Surg. 2015;44:885–8.

Navigation and Guided Surgery

Hani Tohme and Ghida Lawand

1 Introduction

Dental implants have gained traction in replacing missing teeth ever since their introduction into clinical practice. With the increased application of such treatment modalities, it is of great importance to evaluate legitimately the patient's main anatomical landmarks and bone available which is considered imperative in implant placement. This is not to mention providing a proper collaboration between prosthodontists and surgeons to reach successful outcomes [1]. Presurgical planning in both complicated and straightforward cases starts with visual and clinical examination followed by inspecting bone availability using an imaging system [2]. Conventional imaging systems like two-dimensional periapical and panoramic X-rays were often used but are now considered insufficient due to their numerous shortcomings [3]. Distorted and magnified images, superimposed structures, and single image layer view are the reasons why these systems were considered not reliable and led to the introduction of a new technology called the cone beam computed tomography (CBCT) [4]. CBCT is a variation of traditional computed tomography systems that registers data using a cone-shaped X-ray beam to restructure a three-dimensional image of the oral and maxillofacial region. It is used in various applications like orthodontics, endodontics, temporomandibular joint dysfunctions, pathologies, and most importantly in planning endosseous dental implant placement

H. Tohme (✉)
Digital Dentistry Unit, Clinical Director of Postgraduate Program - Removable Prosthodontics Department, Faculty of Dentistry, Saint Joseph University, Beirut, Lebanon
e-mail: hani@tohmeclinic.com

G. Lawand
Prosthodontics and Esthetic Dentistry Department, Faculty of Dentistry, Saint Joseph University, Beirut, Lebanon
e-mail: Ghida.lawand@net.usj.edu.lb

S. A. Parhiz et al. (eds.), *Navigation in Oral and Maxillofacial Surgery*,
https://doi.org/10.1007/978-3-031-06223-0_5

[4]. To improve implant positioning and diminish surgical complications brought by improper planning, the practitioner must have a thorough knowledge of bone width, height, and density so that bone deficiencies or excesses can be evaluated or adjusted prior to implant therapy [5, 6].

Previously, implant placements were freehanded and "surgically driven." This is to say that they mainly hinge on the bone assessed during the surgical procedure which involves a mucoperiosteal flap detachment to obtain adequate visibility. However, currently, the direction has changed towards a more minimally invasive procedure that allows proper implant positioning without any surgical or esthetic compromise and predicts the final result which is also known as "prosthetically driven" implant placement. This is achieved by accurately transferring the wanted treatment plan into the operative field using computer-guided implant surgery [7, 8]. This computer-aided technology has not only assisted the clinician in diagnosing, planning, and treating implant cases with predictable outcomes but also increased patient satisfaction due to the decreased surgical and healing time and reduced invasiveness [9, 10]. Up to the present time, two forms of computer-guided implant surgery systems exist which are the template-based static system and the dynamic navigation system. The first refers to the use of a surgical guide drilling template that determines the direction and depth of the implant bed preparation. The latter uses a stereovision computer triangulation setup that allows the surgeon to visualize in real time the implant site [11].

This chapter summarizes the different computer-guided surgical systems, types of surgical guides, the various software utilized in planning and designing these guides, and the step-by-step workflow for obtaining a successful guided surgery from data acquisition, interpretation, surgical implementation, to prosthesis fabrication with case-based examples. Although this procedure requires extensive experience and knowledge, the chapter provides important remarks and tips for beginners and experts to ensure accurate and reliable implant placement in the exactly planned region.

2 Computer-Guided Implant Surgery Types

There are several types of computer-guided implant surgeries each with its specific indications, advantages, and disadvantages demonstrated in Fig. 1. Knowledge of the following varieties can help the clinician decide which method to follow depending on the clinical situation and the needs of each patient.

Template-Based Static System

Static surgical templates will assist the surgeon in placing the implants just like the planned position. However, the clinician cannot change his planning position while performing the surgery unless the approach is changed into a freehand approach.

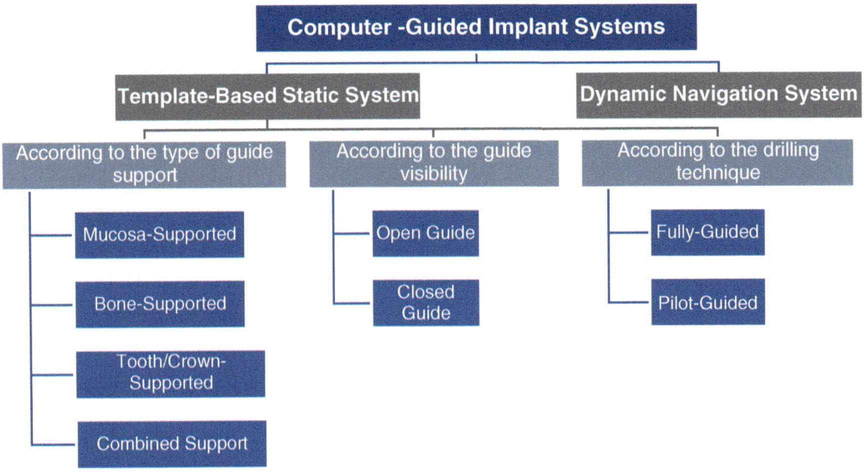

Fig. 1 Diagram representing the different types of computer-guided implant surgery systems (The figure has not been taken from any other published material)

Static templates are classified according to the type of support, guide visibility, and drilling technique.

According to the Type of Support

Mucosa Supported

Mucosa supported guides are usually fabricated in fully edentulous arches. With these guides, the surgery is flapless which means that the clinician cannot visualize the bone present. The guide is often stabilized through the buccal and lingual flanges of the arch. It is also necessary to add fixation pins in a tripod manner to maintain the guide in place. Since the clinician will not open a flap, it is indispensable to punch the gingival areas where the implants will be placed. This is just before the drilling step where punchers usually exist with the guided surgical kit. The advantages of this type of guide lie in the decreased postoperative complications like swelling, pain, and morbidity often caused by flap retraction [12–14]. In addition, this technique is considered more precise than bone-supported guides that usually interfere with the retracted flap [15]. Conversely, this type of template has several disadvantages. This includes the difficulty of guide stabilization in complete edentulous situations in comparison with partially edentulous cases and the inability to perform bone and tissue augmentation procedures. Moreover, this type of guide is contraindicated when there is insufficient keratinized tissue where elevation of a flap is indicated to preserve and reposition existing keratinized tissue around implants [16, 17].

Bone-Supported

This template is made to be supported by bone that is considered to be a more rigid surface than the mucosa. In such guides, a full-thickness flap reflection is necessary and is mainly indicated in cases that need bone augmentation or bone reduction. Bone reduction is recommended when terminal dentition exists where flattening is necessary to place the implants at the same level. A set of sequential guides known as "stackable guides" are fabricated where one is used for bone resection, another for drilling and implant placement, and the last for positioning the provisional restoration. Each guide is pin-indexed to the preceding guide that was fixed to the alveolus with anchor pins [18]. The first guide is fixed according to the patient's bite and often stabilized with a bite index. The main advantage of bone-supported guides is that the practitioner can directly visualize the bone tomography and anatomical structures. He can also perform bone augmentation procedures easily. However, in contrast with flapless techniques, flap retraction can intensify morbidity and postoperative pain leading to decreased patient satisfaction [19–21].

Tooth/Crown-Support Guide

This is when the guide is fully supported by the teeth or crowns present in the patient's mouth. Teeth/crowns are considered rigid structures than are sufficient to stabilize the guide in place and prevent its movement without the need of fixation pins. It is also important to mention that merging DICOM and STL files is considered easier and will result in a more precise guide because there are sufficient reference points that will make it easier for the software to align the files together. In a recent study by Raico Gallardo et al., it was proven that teeth supported guides offer ultimate accuracy in comparison with the aforementioned types [22].

Combined-Support

In cases of partially edentulous arches, the guide fabricated should be maintained on both teeth and soft tissue. This will ensure higher stability than being supported on the mucosa only. In some critical cases where teeth are not enough to hold the template in place or when the teeth are mobile, it is advisable to place fixation anchor pins to ensure that the guide is firm and immobile.

According to Guide Visibility

Open Guide

Open guides allow immediate visibility of the bone and mucosa during drilling through a buccal access formed on the template. Any inaccuracies originating from the planning phase can be easily identified during the surgical procedure preventing

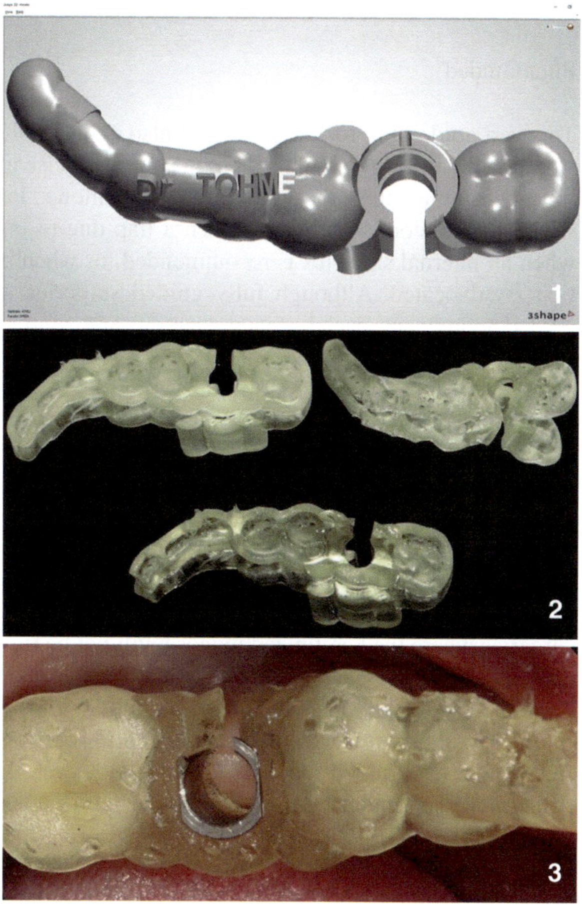

Fig. 2 (1) STL file of the guide with a buccal opening. (2) Printed surgical guide. (3) Intraoral occlusal view of the guide with its sleeve placed intraorally. (With Permission from Dr. Hani Tohme)

any unfortunate event and ensuring correct implant positioning. Also, through this buccal opening, sufficient irrigation is achieved, preventing any overheating (Fig. 2 (1–3)). However, being a less restrictive technique, positioning error may exist which requires more attention [23, 24].

Closed Guide

In this type of guide, the practitioner cannot visualize the bone or the mucosa and cannot see the whole surgical field when performing the implant surgery. In such a case the drills go fully through the template which means that accuracy fully depends on the previous planning and the guide system utilized unlike the open system. Moreover, this system does not allow enough amount of cooling fluid to reach the site which can hinder osseointegration and lead to compromised healing in case overheating occurred [23, 24].

According to the Drilling Technique

Pilot Guided

This is a guide only for the pilot drill also called "pilot drill guide." The clinician would still be working freehand but in a more precise manner and is considered less time consuming than the conventional technique. Pilot drills are recommended when the surgeon is obliged to open a flap due to insufficient keratinized tissue, when an internal sinus lift is recommended, or when bone augmentation or reduction is advocated. Although fully guided surgeries are more accurate than half guided approaches, each has its indications and contraindications [25].

Fully Guided

This type of guide monitors the whole surgical process from the drilling procedure to implant placement. Mostly, fully guided protocols go together with flapless surgeries, taking into account that the presurgical planning and template offer enough information that makes raising a flap unnecessary. However, if inadequate amount of bone or tissues is present, a flap is a prerequisite for performing fully guided surgeries where the keratinized mucosa will not be influenced by punching and the surgeon can easily place bone substitutes. Fully guided surgeries proved to offer optimum accuracy in many randomized clinical trials when comparing the planned implant position to the executed results. It also showed minimum error compared to freehand or half guided surgeries [26–28]. However, this is the most expensive and delicate type of guides because it highly relies on fidelity and any error can lead to wrong implant position [29].

Dynamic Navigation System

This technique is also referred to as navigation-guided surgery and involves 3D planning with cone beam computed tomograph (CBCT) exploration, and prosthetic analysis before the surgical procedure. A guided template is not used during the surgery, while with special instruments and specific software, bone drilling and implant placement are completely tracked with the navigation system. The patient's anatomy and the surgical procedures are shown in real time in a 3D software application. The system is constituted of a technology called stereovision and supported with natural light cameras and includes a patient jaw attachment and a handpiece attachment [29]. This provides real motion tracking effect of the surgery. The navigation systems commonly used are DenX Image Guided Implantology, X-Guide Dynamic 3D Navigation, Navident, and Inliant [30]. This approach is considered advantageous compared to the static option because the surgeon is able to interfere instantly while performing the surgery and change implant direction relative to the anatomical structures available as well as the implant size [31]. On the other hand, this method is scarcely applied compared to the template-based method for several reasons. First, an inaccuracy in the navigation system can influence the spatial correlation between the points of reference and the real anatomical structures in the patient's mouth leading to misinterpretation and a faulty drilling protocol which is also echoed in implant placement [32]. For inexperienced dentists, the iatrogenic consequences of this technique are high which requires thorough knowledge and practice before being applied on a patient. This procedure is also considered highly expensive compared to the static guide as it requires a special technology [33]. Moreover, clinical studies on its efficiency and reliability are still insufficient to evaluate its advantages and compare it with other methods [34, 35].

Image-to-Patient Registration in Dynamic Navigation System

The patient's picture coordinates and physical space coordinates must be linked, a process known as registration, before navigation is possible [29, 30]. The coordinates of corresponding artificial or anatomical (fiducial) points are identified in the paired-point technique, and the geometrical transformation that best aligns these points is computed. With the use of a localizer probe from the navigation system, the correct points are identified in the picture data and shown on the patient. Bone markers, which are invasively fixed to the patient's frontal bone or alveolar process, are the most reliable procedure and the gold standard. These markers should not be left in place for an extended amount of time because they are intrusive, necessitate extra surgery, may infect, and may cause patient discomfort [29, 30]. Thus, noninvasive methods have been investigated. Fiducial markers may be included on denture-fixed radiography scan templates to use as registration templates. A scan prosthesis or a vacuum mouthpiece may also be installed with external registration frames (jaw-around frames with fiducials).

With mean target registration errors of 0.93–0.94 mm for all three approaches, registration templates or external registration frames may, under ideal circumstances, give registration accuracy comparable to that of bone markers [30–35]. The repositioning process for registration templates, however, can result in misplaced or improperly fitting templates. The robustness of the oral mucosa in edentulous patients prevents the stable and invariant positioning of registration templates or external registration frames. The issue might be effectively overcome by using three miniscrews and an adaptor sphere to attach the template to the underlying bone using a fixed-reference approach [30–35].

Surgical Navigation in Dynamic Navigation System

The navigation system is prepared for use during surgery after registration [30]. The stereoscopic camera must continually record the tracked surgical drill and the dynamic reference frame. Special guided views, which are displayed on a computer screen or using head-mounted equipment, assist in locating the planned implant's location and tracing its course into the bone. The accuracy of the drill's position and angulations are indicated by the navigation software, but the surgeon's physical dexterity is still required for the actual drilling.

The procedure is described by first scanning the patient and any external registration frames, bone markers, or scan prosthesis/registration templates. Second, use a software tool to plan the placement of the implant. After that, using registration templates, external registration frames, or bone markers, register the image to the patient in step 3. Finally, drilling is performed where the drill navigation is in accordance with the predetermined surgical strategy [30].

Compared to unguided manual insertion, surgical navigation enables an extremely substantial improvement in drilling accuracy. There were no statistically significant differences between the two surgical navigation systems and computer-guided stereolithographic surgical templates. Mean lateral errors of 0.7–0.8 mm (maximum: 1.6–2 mm) for the implant shoulder and 1.0–1.2 mm (maximum: 2.4–3.4 mm) for the implant apex were observed in a prospective, randomized clinical comparison of two navigation systems. Oral implant surgery has been successfully applied in both partial and total edentulous patients, flapless techniques, challenging anatomical conditions, and following tumor surgery [30–35].

Dynamic guiding has shown to be a useful tool in a variety of surgical operations, including zygoma implant surgery, the removal of tumors and foreign bodies, orthognathic and reconstructive surgery, temporomandibular joint surgery, skull base surgery, as well as for education and training [30–35].

Surgical Template Fabrication Using Navigation Systems

The creation of surgical templates can also be done using surgical navigation systems. Instead of using the patient, the navigation operation is carried out in the lab on the registered dental stone cast of the patient. The base plate of the lab setup can be simply mounted with the dynamic reference frame. Because the wax-up may be identified using the navigation probe on the dental stone cast, a scan prosthesis may not be required. A stereotactic targeting device is used, as opposed to dynamic guidance of the tracked drill. A tracked, adjustable mechanical arm with six degrees of freedom that is aligned with the intended trajectory and enables stiff drill guidance using the best method is the stereotactic targeting device.

The stereotactic targeting device is used to drill the dental stone cast in order to provide a surgical guide. The surgical bur tubes are then placed by inserting metal rods into the stereotactic drill holes. In one dental laboratory session, the bur tubes are bonded into a resin template. Alternately, a metal rod advanced through the stereotactic targeting device may be used to position a surgical bur tube on the dental stone casts, and then a prefabricated template may be polymerized using an ultraviolet light-curing resin.

Significance of Each Method

In some clinical circumstances, either approach will be preferable to the freehand approach. The clinician's preference and prior expertise will determine whether to use static or dynamic navigation. So, the following can be accomplished using any navigation technique [30–35]:

1. The practitioner wants to employ a flapless method to prevent upsetting the superficial section of the graft by elevating a flap because the site has already undergone ridge augmentation.
2. Using a navigation system will ensure suitable spacing of the implants from the teeth and give accuracy in maintaining the right space between the implants when installation of adjacent implants demands exact spacing between the implants and adjacent teeth.
3. When precise implant angulation is necessary, which is crucial in the esthetic zone and for prostheses that are screw-retained.
4. To manage the placement's depth.
   (a) To prevent nerve injury.
   (b) To elevate the sinus floor through the implant preparation site while positioning the preparatory osteotomy next to the sinus floor.
   (c) To consciously engage the sinus or nasal floor to stabilize the bicortical implant.

For edentulous instances, a static guide created by a CT scan is advised. Since intrabony fiducial markers cannot yet be used in navigation systems, dynamic navigation necessitates registration of the jaw to the navigation system. When a flapless technique is desired, when implant placement is crucial for a planned full arch fixed crown and bridge type prosthesis, when the clinician wants to use a bone reduction guide to accurately provide space for the planned prosthesis, and when the guide can help in preoperatively fabricating a provisional prosthesis on models created from the static guide itself, a static CT-generated guide should be used for edentulous cases [28, 29]. However, dynamic navigation is recommended when the patient has a small mouth opening, when it is challenging to see directly, when ideal implant placement will be hampered by the presence of nearby natural teeth, when the implant is to be placed the same day as the CBCT scan, and when it is difficult to access areas like a second molar [30–35].

Which approach will work best in a given circumstance will be obvious. Because of the time- and money-effective workflow, the use of the dynamic approach may become more prevalent as the clinician's experience and surgical proficiency grow. Dynamic navigation needs teeth in dentate individuals to stabilize the registration clip and array [30–35]. On mobile teeth or temporarily cemented provisional restorations, the registration and clip array should not be used. Additionally, patients with a small mouth opening or crestal bone loss may need drill extenders to insert implants in molar areas that are difficult to see directly. Accurate spacing between the implants and the neighboring teeth is necessary when placing adjacent implants.

Table 1 This table summarizes the parameters evaluated in dynamic and static guided surgery (The table has not been taken from any other published material)

Parameters evaluated	Static guidance	Dynamic guidance
CBCT guided	Yes	Yes
Flapless	Yes	Yes
Need for dental scan	Yes	No
Spatial limitations	Yes	No
Specific surgical kit	Yes	No
Time for guide fabrication	Yes	No
Alter surgical plan	No	Yes
Surgical time	Shorter	Longer
Planning software	Comprehensive	Simple
Clinical application	Dentate/edentulous	Dentate/edentulous

Both static and dynamic systems may be employed; the choice will, however, depend on the clinical expertise and particular case factors. Because dynamic navigation is adaptable, the clinician is free to modify the surgical strategy as needed [28–35]. Additionally, since no laboratory work is needed, instant scanning, planning, and guidance can be provided the same day a patient presents. The physician needs to be aware that proficiency requires a learning curve. For training, simulation, and manikin practice, more time may be needed.

The parameters evaluated in each technique is summarized in the table below (Table 1).

3 Workflow and Requirements of Computer-Guided Implant Surgery

Prosthetic and Surgical Planning

CBCT

The most important part of guided surgery is to have images with a quality that is appropriate for diagnostic assessment. As mentioned earlier, the most reliable computed tomography imaging technique for implantology is the CBCT. This technique uses either cone or pyramid shaped divergent X-rays that rotate around the area to be captured and are able to detect complete volume of images [36]. Several models of CBCT machines exist in the market and its tools are numerous. Their classification is mainly based on the field of image to be captured also known as the "field of view" or "FOV" that can be large, medium, or small. In order to choose which type suits the case best, the FOV should be chosen slightly greater than the anatomical area of interest to include regions that might be affected during implant placement and for that it is always advisable to capture the field that is covering the whole arch [37]. The recommended ratio by the American Academy of Oral and Maxillofacial Radiology in dental implantology for FOV is 10 × 5 for each of the lower or upper arch and 10 × 10 for the upper and lower arches [38]. In order to obtain a precise image, several recommendations exist for optimizing the results. First, the patient should remove any metal parts like earrings, jewelry, hairclips, or denture with metallic framework that may interfere with the X-rays and lead to artifacts. Second, the CBCT must be captured in an open-mouth situation. This is important when planning prosthetically driven implants so that the occlusal surface of the opposing arch would not interfere with the planning process. For doing so, the patient should bite on cotton rolls ensuring that the upper arch is away from the lower arch. In cases of complete or severe partially edentulous cases, it is advisable to perform a CBCT using a radiological template. This template should demonstrate the appropriate position of teeth with radiopaque markers that will help the dentist plan a prosthetically driven implant position. In such cases the radiographic template must be stabilized in the mouth using a silicone bite index to prevent its movement and to make sure that it precisely adheres to the gums without any airspace. Also, an index is required in cases of dentate patients with severe deep bite when a cotton roll does not ensure disocclusion of both arches. Another tip that may help obtain an accurate file is to place cotton rolls in the sulcus to separate the cheeks and lips during the imaging process. The patient is also advised not to make his tongue touch the palate and not to move or swallow when performing the image. It is very important to note that changes in the mucosa and alveolar bone during the time between the presurgical evaluation and the surgery have to be taken into consideration. Inadequate planning may result from alveolar ridge resorption and changes in the thickness of soft tissue due to recent teeth extraction that will also not appear clearly on the CBCT. After the image is obtained, the file is exported in the Digital Imaging and Communications in Medicine (DICOM) uncompressed format and burnt on a CD or sent through a platform called "WeTransfer" [39].

Radiographic template requirements when performing a CBCT:

The radiographic template used in complete edentulous patients can either be made of the existing denture of the patient or of a transparent acrylic that is a duplicate of an existing or a newly fabricated denture. In case of using his existing denture, the first important step to make sure of is that the denture is in intimate contact with the soft tissues and that it is esthetically pleasing [15]. This is crucial because planning the prosthetically driven implants will be according to teeth position. If the denture is esthetically acceptable but does not adhere sufficiently to the underlying tissues, the denture should be relined first. Airspace should not be visible between the denture and the soft tissues. In addition, it is important to make sure that the denture is thick enough to be able to differentiate between the acrylic borders and air or else holes will be visible in the scanned prosthesis and should be devoid of any metallic framework that will interfere with the CBCT taken and create artifacts [15]. The template should have a minimum of 6–8 round convex radiopaque markers with a size of 2–3 mm positioned on the vestibule and the palate. The more are the radiographic markers the better since this will speed up the superimposition process in later steps. The markers should not be present on the occlusal surface of the teeth because the occlusal surface is one of the important regions that guide the practitioner to positioning the implant in a prosthetically driven scenario which means that this area should be clear and well demarcated. The markers are made of gutta percha, glass beads, or composite resin. Some authors recommended the use of pre-installed markers such as mini-implants that can increase the accuracy of the scan prosthesis matching process and later the positioning of the guide [40].

Digital Impression

In order to be able to perform a guided surgery, a digital model should be initiated. This digital model can be formed either from an intraoral scanner, direct scanning of a silicone impression using a desktop scanner, or scanning a poured plaster model using a desktop scanner. Choosing which method depends on the clinical situation. Intraoral scanners offer accurate files in cases where enough teeth exist in the arch where it is easy for the clinician to superimpose STL and DICOM files. However, in cases of edentulous arches or distal free end Kennedy Class I cases, it is often indicated to take a classical impression followed by creating a virtual model due to the decreased accuracy of intraoral scanners in such situations. However, in a study by Nagata et al. who compared silicone and digital impression method for mandibular free end situations, results show that intraoral scanners provide a more accurate implant surgery [41].

Planning Software

Various software exist for planning implant placement all of which have the same basic principles but differ in the additional features each of them offers. The clinician will decide on the planning platform that meets his needs as his choice will depend on the type of implants he uses, the type of guide, and the complexity of the case. Examples of the implant planning software programs include coDiagnostiX by Dental Wings, Implant Studio by 3Shape, Blue Sky Plan by Blue Sky Bio, and NobelClinician by Nobel Biocare. Some other proprietary CBCT software offer treatment planning options like NewTom implant planning software and Galileos by Sirona Dental System [42]. The computer software permits the user to utilize the DICOM data obtained from the CBCT for interpretation and representation of bone densities and volumes prior to the surgical procedure. Although bone density is a relative measurement that relies on the gray values of the image, machine tuning, and software analysis, it is often important when planning for immediate implant placement. This is because it allows the surgeon to expect if he can achieve a high insertion torque and ensure primary stability or not. Some software like coDiagnostix allows for the visualization of implant abutments along with the implant body which is necessary when placing angulated implants in full-arch situations like All-on-four. This also allows the clinician to modify the implant inclination and gingival height according to how he visualizes the final predictable restorative result. Having software with many integrated specifications will allow for a more legitimate computer-guided implant surgery with an ideal surgical and prosthetic implant position. Planning implant placement involves several steps that may have a different sequence in each of the programs listed previously but generally follow a similar workflow. The steps of this workflow are demonstrated in Table 2.

Table 2 This table summarizes the workflow of planning implant placement (The table has not been taken from any other published material)

Steps for planning implant placement
(a) Importing DICOM and STL files
(b) Drawing the panoramic curve
(c) Drawing left and right nerve canals in mandibular arch
(d) Segmentation
(e) Choosing the appropriate implant size, position, and angulation

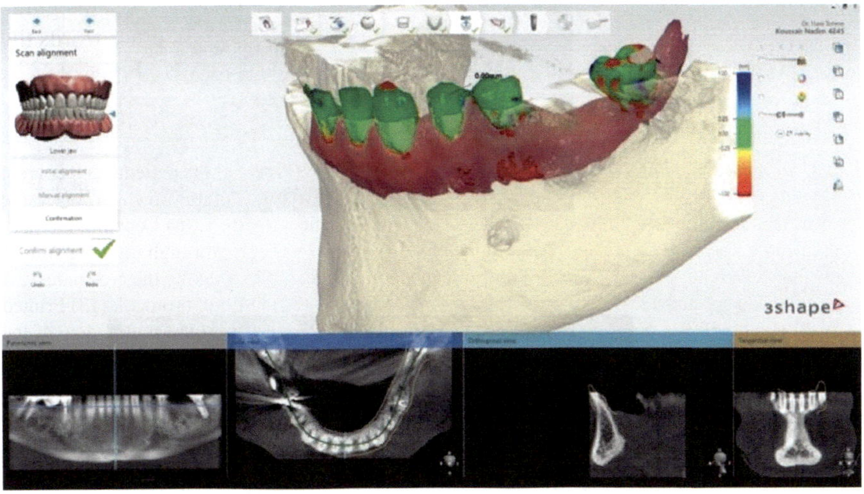

Fig. 3 STL file superimposed over the DICOM file. A colorimetric map is available in order to determine how accurate the superimposition is. Green color indicates the lowest deviation. (With Permission from Dr. Hani Tohme)

Importing DICOM and STL Files

These two files are the building blocks of guided surgery. CBCT DICOM files do not demonstrate soft tissue and teeth precisely which necessitate merging an STL file obtained from intraorally scanning the needed region and superimposing it with the DICOM file having teeth as reference points (Fig. 3). Once the DICOM and STL data are merged, the clinician can now plan his prosthetically driven restoration. The CAD software generally provides a smile library with many forms and shapes to design the missing teeth and allow a proper teeth setup. Another way for doing this instead of a virtual wax up is performing a conventional wax up, scanning the model, and integrating the STL file with the dataset which requires additional time.

Drawing the Panoramic Curve

This is the curve determined when the appropriate horizontal section is determined and this is when the ridge is completely visible (Fig. 4). Delineating the panoramic curve is done by connecting points together generally located in the center. This is

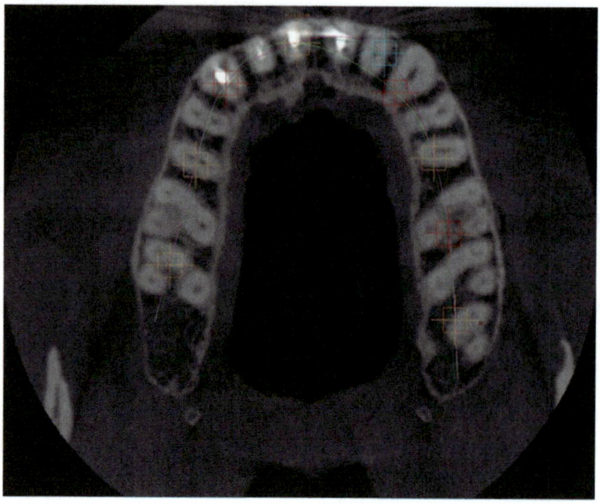

Fig. 4 A drawing of the panoramic curve (With Permission from Dr. Hani Tohme)

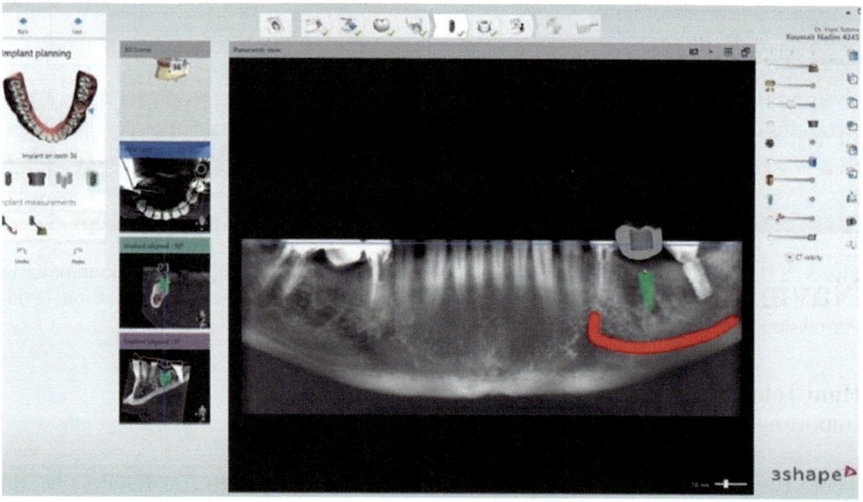

Fig. 5 Left inferior nerve canal delineated in red. (With Permission from Dr. Hani Tohme)

important to make sure that the implant is placed on the crest of the ridge with the appropriate bone borders.

Mapping Nerve Canals in Mandibular Arch

Since the inferior alveolar canal is one of the most important anatomical landmarks to take into account when performing an implant surgery in the lower arch, mapping its trajectory is indispensable (Fig. 5) [42]. This step should be done carefully as the clinician can scroll through the different cuts to determine the nerve from its origin to its insertion. This is delicate because an anterior loop may exist in the mental nerve region and cannot be visible to the clinician if not drawn. The software can automatically determine how close the implant is to the nerve, giving a warning sign if the distance was less than 2 mm. Some programs automatically trace the whole canal using specific algorithms determined by comparing the gray level densities and can be then adjusted by the practitioner. However, in cases where artifacts exist or the patient is osteopenic, it is hard to delineate the borders of the nerve [43].

Segmentation

The segmentation tool present in some planning software allows the clinician to manipulate the 3-dimensional volumes in order to create clearer hyper-spectral models. Artifacts and scatters produced from metallic restorations that interfere with the visualization of the implant location in 3D can be trimmed with care making it easier for the clinician to plan but cannot be disregarded from the two-dimensional image. In addition, the user can create layers or masks (teeth alone, teeth, and the ridge) giving each a color and separate regions from surrounding structures (Fig. 6). These layers can be turned on and off according to the step being performed making the clinician understand better the structures present. In some programs, there is the transparency option that allows the handler to see some structures transparent and underlying structures opaquer [42]. Manual segmentation is well-thought-out as time consuming and it is hard sometimes for the dentist himself to target specific structures which made researchers start working on automatic image segmentation technologies.

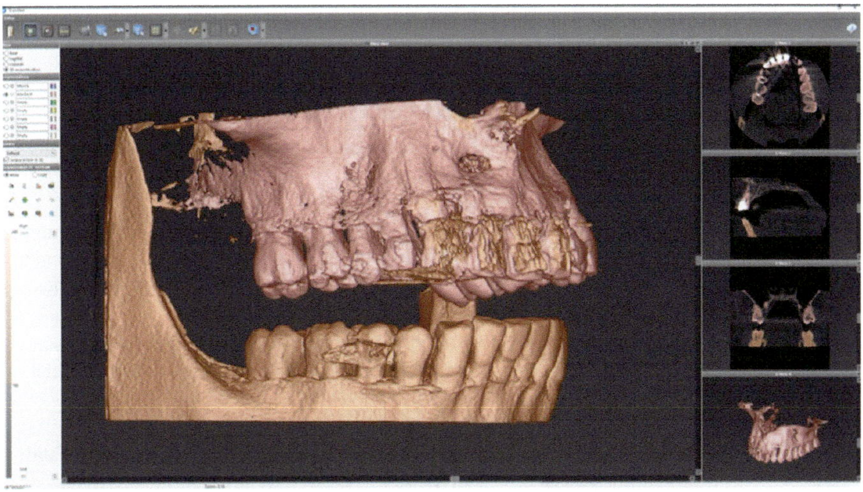

Fig. 6 Maxillary arch segmented in light pink color removing all the artifacts caused by metallic restorations. (With Permission from Dr. Hani Tohme)

Choosing the Appropriate Implant Size, Position, and Angulation

1. Anatomical Considerations during planning:

   The sequence of positioning the implant in place starts by defining the anatomical landmarks that are close to the site of implant placement. This includes all the nerves, blood vessels, teeth, teeth roots, implants, as well as bone contours, density, and volume.

   (a) Nerve/Blood Vessels/Sinus

   In scenarios where there is nerve or sinus proximity, implants are most precisely positioned with a computed guided template. This will decrease the possibility of patient morbidity and will ensure a safe surgical procedure. Table 3 summarizes all the nerves/vessels/sinuses present in the anterior or posterior region of the upper and lower arches and lists the limitations and complications if these structures were violated.

   (b) Teeth/Teeth Roots

   Placing single or multiple implants within the dental arch is demanding considering the closeness to adjacent tooth roots which necessitate falling within specific outlined guidelines and recommendations [50–53]. The distance between an implant and a tooth is 1.5 mm and 3 mm between two implants [51, 54]. Most of the software used for planning guided surgeries tend to isolate teeth along with their roots next to the edentulous region according to their sensitivity to Hounsfield to allow proper placement of implant in the appropriate planned area. Some other software allow the user to draw lines to delineate teeth roots. This is often important when the implants are to be placed in edentulous areas with root proximity or in cases

Table 3 This table lists all the anatomical landmarks that should be taken care of when planning for implant placement (The table has not been taken from any other published material)

Arch	Region	Nerves /blood vessels	Complications and limitations
Maxilla	Anterior region	Nasopalatine canal and foramen	Limits the vertical height possible for implant sites [44]
	Posterior region	Maxillary sinus	Perforation of the Schneiderian membrane during sinus floor elevation or during implant placement or displacement of implants into the maxillary sinus [45]
Mandible	Anterior region	1. Anterior loop	Presence of symmetric anterior loops can be as frequent as 76% to 88% and its violation can lead to paresthesia of anterior mandibular teeth [46]
		2. Median lingual vascular	Violations of this canal can lead to serious hemorrhagic scenarios and can sometimes be fatal [47, 48].
	Posterior region	Inferior alveolar nerve	Violation leads to permanent paresthesia of that side of the patient's jaw, teeth, and lips [49]

of excessively convergent or divergent roots. Challenging clinical situations like placing implants in tight spaces with a minimum leeway of bone go through some surgical dilemmas that cannot be implemented by the free-hand technique. The planning software allow the clinician to first visualize the virtual analog of the proposed implant in place. He can also use the parallelism tool that will help him make the placed implant as parallel as possible to adjacent implants or teeth. This will allow him to decide on the appropriate implant size and diameter. Moreover, enough inter-implant or tooth-implant distance must be determined in order to place the sleeves in the surgical guide with adequate material to avoid breakage of the guide.

(c) Bone contours/density/volume

Several bone boundaries exist in the maxillary and mandibular arches that the dentist should take into consideration. The preliminary bone contour boundary is the buccolingual width of the alveolar bone in the site of implant placement. The second bone contour boundary is the distance from the alveolar crest till the basal bone that will determine the vertical height of implant bed preparation. This is important to ensure that sufficient bone exists in the coronal, middle, and apical regions. It is also important to mention that facial or lingual concavities do exist and implant position must be changed accordingly. When the user positions the virtual implant, a safety margin appears that is usually adjusted to be 2 mm [55]. The planning program will alarm the user if these boundaries are violated by changing the color of the implant from green to red. Some software also permits the user to act out bone augmentation measures. With this facility one can estimate how much volume is needed for grafting and where the fixation or tenting screws can be positioned. Moreover, the user can also see bone density which is important in case he is planning for immediate implant placement to make sure that primary stability does exist. Because of the nature of CBCT imaging, these measurements are not accurate.

2. Restorative considerations during planning:

The fundamental purpose of placing implants is the final prosthetic result and this is why the clinician should have a restorative-driven mind-set. Communication between the surgeon, prosthodontist, and lab technician is necessary to achieve the wanted results. The restorability of implants depends on several factors which can be evaluated on the CBCT. It is important to evaluate the inter-arch space meaning the relation of the edentulous region with the opposing arch in order to determine if enough room is available for the implant to be restored. This is critical because it is a normal physiological process to have the opposing teeth creep into the edentulous space. This assessment is not always guaranteed on a CBCT because the field of view may only include the region to be restored and the opposing dentition may be disregarded. This is serious when choosing the appropriate abutment design on the planning software taking into account the crown inclination that if exaggerated may lead to biological and mechanical problems [56]. It is also important to evaluate the mesiodistal distance available to restore the implant with all the esthetic considerations of having an appropriate papilla height and a good emergence.

In case of multiple implants in an edentulous arch, supreme implant placement is recommended so restorative evaluation is highly important. First, the restorative space must be respected following the appropriate occlusal plane, the bearing hard and soft tissues of the edentulous ridge, and the orofacial structures [8, 12, 16, 27]. According to this, the practitioner can know what treatment plan he should follow. For instance, if the space between the implant and the incisal edge of the tooth is more than 15 mm, a hybrid prosthesis is recommended. In case of severe maxillary atrophy with decreased lip support, an overdenture is needed having the space between the implant and the incisal edge 9–11 mm. In situations of tooth-only defect, the type of prosthesis should be porcelain fused to metal. In order to facilitate edentulous implant reconstruction cases, specific strategic implant positions are recommended including the canines, first premolars, and molars. In addition, some investigators advocate that in the maxillary arch, the central incisors are also strategic positions. For instance, in all four cases, the implants must be placed in the following sites: two anterior implants in the lateral incisor region and two posterior implants in the second premolar region.

Using this information, the practitioner can quantify the extent of prosthetic space either by measuring the distance between the intaglio of the denture and the incisal edge using a caliper. During this initial assessment of a patient's dental prosthesis, estimates can be made regarding potential alveolar ridge reduction to expand the amount of prosthetic space for the final prosthetic restoration. Surgical templates for bone reduction (stackable guides) will guide the surgeon for the appropriate amount of bone reduction required prior to implant placement. This reduction permits an increase in the amount of restorative space needed once the implant body is in place. This anticipated treatment course is only conceivable with high attentiveness to the preoperative implant-site evaluation and treatment plan, using implant planning software programs [42].

Surgical Guide Designation

The design of the guide is influenced by many factors including the arch (maxillary or mandibular), type of support (mucosa, bone, teeth, or combined), number of implants and their location, software facilities, production technology (subtractive/additive), type of fixation (screws/pins), and indication (immediate loading, requires bone reduction). The design of the guide is very subjective and relative to each practitioner's experience where each can make a different design of the same case. The user can manipulate the software to reach the needed criteria and also add bars or tubes for cross-arch stabilization and increasing the rigidity of the guide. Another important note to mention is that after the surgeon starts with drilling, upon completion of the first implant bed preparation, he can add a fixation pin in the site of preparation to stabilize the guide further. After designing the guide, the user is asked to accept the planned implant position with the surgical guide design so that the practitioner can proceed to exporting the 3D model of the guide in an STL format. Upon exporting the guide, the user can also export the drilling protocol along with the surgical report. The drilling protocol sequence is highly important to follow in order to reach the desired result.

Surgical Guide Fabrication

With the introduction of CAD-CAM technology, surgical guides are currently produced either using subtractive manufacturing by milling or additive manufacturing by printing, the latter being the most common. Milled guides are highly accurate but are expensive and complex in construction. In addition, offset parameter settings must be identified in order not to create tight guides. Henprasert et al. compared additive and subtractive techniques and found no difference in terms of accuracy but printing technologies are easier in fabrication, offer lower costs, produce less waste, and have a reduced laboratory time. Thereby, additive manufacturing is gaining popularity rapidly in dentistry [57, 58]. The production sequence is as follows (Table 4):

There are many printing methodologies available in the market such as SLA, DLP, and Polyjet. The manufacturing procedures of all technologies are alike but can produce different outcomes. The SLA technology known as stereolithography is a fast-prototyping technology that relies on UV laser beams projected through X and Y scanning mirrors for solidifying the liquid photopolymerizing resin and transforming it into a hard 3D object. Following polymerization, it is suggested to immerse the printed model into a chemical bath to clean the model post-printing. PolyJet technology, however, uses a jetting process where small droplets called voxels are spurted into a platform then cured using UV light. This technology considered to be the most advanced one in 3D printing provides a very smooth surface due to its microscopic layer resolution with an accuracy of 16 microns. Examples of this 3D printing device are the Stratasys which are the only printers used in the dental field that function in a triple injectable technology. Finally, digital light processing (DLP) technology is similar to SLA printing except that traditional light source instead of UV light is used in order to harden the resin [60]. Various researches evaluated the accuracy of each printing machinery, concerning the capability to reconstruct the virtual 3D models into the exact physical surgical guides [61–64]. In

Table 4 This table lists all the steps for surgical guide production. (The table has not been taken from any other published material)

Steps for surgical guide production (additive technique) [59]
1. Finalizing the surgical guide design to create a 3D virtual model using a CAD software
2. Exporting the design in an STL format for production
3. File is converted to slices of equal thickness (uniform layer height)
4. 3D printer proceeds in printing the guide from the bottom to the top slice by slice
5. Guide post-processing by curing and polishing
6. Disinfection

guided implantology, measuring accuracy involves calculating the angular distortion, the point of entry deviation, and the position of implant apex compared to the planned one. These are influenced by several factors involved during printing which include layer thickness, orientation, shape of the model, quality of the material, type of printer used, and software used to virtually design the model [65]. Anunmana et al. compared the 3 types of additive printing technology to evaluate the most accurate technology in producing guides with the most exact implant positions. Results show that PolyJet had the best outcome regarding the 3D deviations at the entry point and at the apex, meanwhile, the DLP printer had the shortest processing time [66]. The last step is disinfecting the surgical guide. Sterilizing the guides must be done using ethylene oxide gas. Decontamination of the surgical guide using chlorohexidine gluconate was not considered efficient. Disinfection can also be done but using 70% of ethanol for 15 minutes [67].

4 Limitations of Computer-Guided Implant Surgery

There are several shortcomings of a guided surgery that still make some practitioners avoid it. First, it is considered a lengthy procedure as it requires more time presurgically than the traditional method. Second, this protocol necessitates extra costs including the 3D imaging system, the planning software used, the guided surgical drilling kit, and the printed surgical guide which adds a lot to the cost estimate given to the patient [68, 69]. Third, just like all new technologies, beginners in the field are on a steep learning curve due to the high amount of experience and skills it involves not only for the surgeon and technician but also for the whole dental team [70]. However, in a recent study by Cassetta et al., it was proven that the static guided surgery has no learning curve effect which makes the dentist able to insert the implant in the correct position without being affected by his own experience [71]. Moreover, this technique brings an increased risk compared to open flap freehand approaches because of the invisibility and lack of tactile control [72]. In addition, because of the surgical guide intimate contact with the tissues, cooling irrigation might not reach the implant bed site while drilling that may cause bone overheating. Although osteotomy preparation using a template induced higher bone temperatures than conventional approaches, the temperature reached was still considered safe to the bone and would not impede the osseointegration process. Consequently, ample amount of irrigation should be provided during the drilling process when a guide is present to alleviate thermal incidences in the presence of a guide [73].

5 Common Mistakes Encountered in Guided Surgery

Accuracy is crucial when doing a guided surgery and any deviation can lead to unmatched results between the planned and the placed implant. This is often considered dangerous when the case is very delicate in terms of bone availability or implant proximity to anatomical structures. Computer-guided surgery involves a series of diagnostic and surgical episodes, and error can creep in at any phase of treatment that demand mastering each step of the workflow. Thus, inaccuracies may result from one or many errors that clinicians should steer clear of. These errors include:

1. Wrong acquisition of the tomographic and intraoral image and data processing [74]. These errors include spatial resolution issues, superimposition methods, scanned data, and programs utilized. In order to obtain optimum registration of both DICOM and STL files, the previous recommendations listed in the requirements section should be followed. Artifacts, limited field of view, distorted image due to patient's movement, voxel size, and scan strategy applied can all play major roles in the clinical accuracy and can affect data merging [37, 75–78].
2. Unstable guide due to wrong positioning or its movement while drilling that leads to displacement when placing the implants [79–81].
3. Manufacturing error due to the technology utilized [82]. This depends on whether the guide is printed or milled. Accuracy of the additive fabrication was found to be ranging from 0.1 to 0.5 mm based on recent research which was found to be clinically acceptable [83]. Although it is not the popular method, subtractive manufacturing was proven to be superior in terms of accuracy compared to additive technology [84].
4. Reduced mouth opening that displaces the surgical instruments during bone perforation leading to incorrect angulation of the drills during perforation causing lateral deviation. This is why one of the main contraindications of guided surgery is a patient with limited mouth opening [85–87].
5. Deviation from the planned axis of insertion may occur in partially guided procedures that involve a pilot drill or those where drilling stops before implant placement. This deviation is due to the fact that implants usually have an affinity to follow the path with the least resistance [27]. Principally in cases having a soft bone type deviations are most likely to occur.
6. Error due to the mechanical tolerance of the surgical instruments or what is known as bur cylinder gap. For example, one of the systems has a 5 mm long guiding sleeves with an internal diameter of 0.15–0.20 mm bigger than the respective bur. This tolerance permits a theoretical angular distortion of around 2.29 degrees which, at a hypothetical distance of 20 mm from the cylinder, leads to a lateral deviation of 1 mm approximately [88]. These calculations cannot be generalized to other systems, because each has different tolerances between drills and guiding cylinders.

Studies have shown that it was more common to find a big vertical error than a large horizontal fault. This may be attributed to that alveolar bone superior border is difficult to differentiate in CT data during the implant planning [69]. Subsequently, after implant positioning, some cases may need a little profounder placement after removing the guide [86]. The reports of the fifth ITI consensus conference on computer-guided surgery showed an inaccuracy at the implant entry point of, on average, 1.12 mm and an apex inaccuracy around 1.39 mm with a mean angular deviation of 3.9 degrees [40]. Because of this, virtual planning should be done judiciously, with a correct safety margin secured to avoid damaging the vital structures.

6 Guided Single Implants

Guided surgeries for single implant placements are often considered easier than multiple implant cases since they require less pre-planning steps. However, difficulties still exist. For example, in cases of tooth/root proximity, it is hard for the surgeon to plan the implant position or design the guide. Two cases are demonstrated to explain in detail the workflow of single implant guided surgery passing through all the steps from diagnosis to restoration.

Case 1: Immediate Guided Implant Placement with Immediate Loading

Patient appeared at the clinic with a non-restorable lower premolar. Clinical examination (Fig. 7 (1, 2)) was made first to determine the contour of the bone present, the quality and quantity of mucosa, the mesiodistal distance, inter-arch space, and the occlusal status of the patient. The occlusal status is highly important in this case because implant placement is planned to be immediate followed by immediate loading. This means that if the patient had parafunctional habits, overloading the implant instantly would lead to its failure. Following the clinical examination, scans were made for the upper and lower arches followed by a bite scan (Fig. 7 (3)). This scan is highly important in order to design the immediate temporary for the patient and to superimpose it on the DICOM file obtained from the CBCT (Fig. 7 (4–6)). Following this, the user has to start planning for the implant position, implant type, length, and diameter. In immediate cases, it is always advisable to place the implant 2 mm below the tooth root to gain primary stability. Moreover, it is often recommended to follow an undersized drilling protocol in order to create an osteotomy that is narrower than the actual planned implant bed size. This will ensure implant placement with a high insertion torque [89]. In addition, implant angulation must be prosthetically driven

Fig. 7 (1) Premolar frontal view. (2) Premolar occlusal view. (3) Upper, lower, and bite scan taken by Trios intraoral scanner. (4) Trimming the existing crown. (5) Facial view of the designed temporary restoration. (6) Occlusal view of the designed temporary crown. (7) Implant position from the panoramic cut. (8) Sagittal implant cut. (9) Implant position in relation to the panoramic curve. (10) Implant position from an axial view. (11) Implant planning on the planning software called Implant Studio. (12 and 13) Lateral view of the guide design. (14) Implant position from different views. (15) Occlusal surface of the guide design. (16) Drilling protocol of the planned implant. (17) Printed surgical guide without sleeve. (18) Printed surgical guide with sleeve. (19) Milled temporary crown with titanium base. (20) Intraoral view of the surgical guide. (21–24) Drilling sequence. (25) Occlusal view of implant position. (26) Occlusal view of the temporary restoration. (27) Periapical X-ray of the implant with the titanium base immediately after surgery. (28) Emergence profile of the gum after healing phase. (29) Intraoral scans of the emergence profile, implant position using the scan body, opposing arch, and bite registration. (30) Final screw retained crown with the titanium base (Variobase by Straumann). (31) Access hole of the final prosthesis placed in the middle of the occlusal surface signifying the importance of a prosthetically driven guided surgery. (32) Occlusal view of the final restoration. (33) Palatal view of the final restoration. (34) Periapical X-ray of the implant with the final prosthesis. (With Permission from Dr. Hani Tohme)

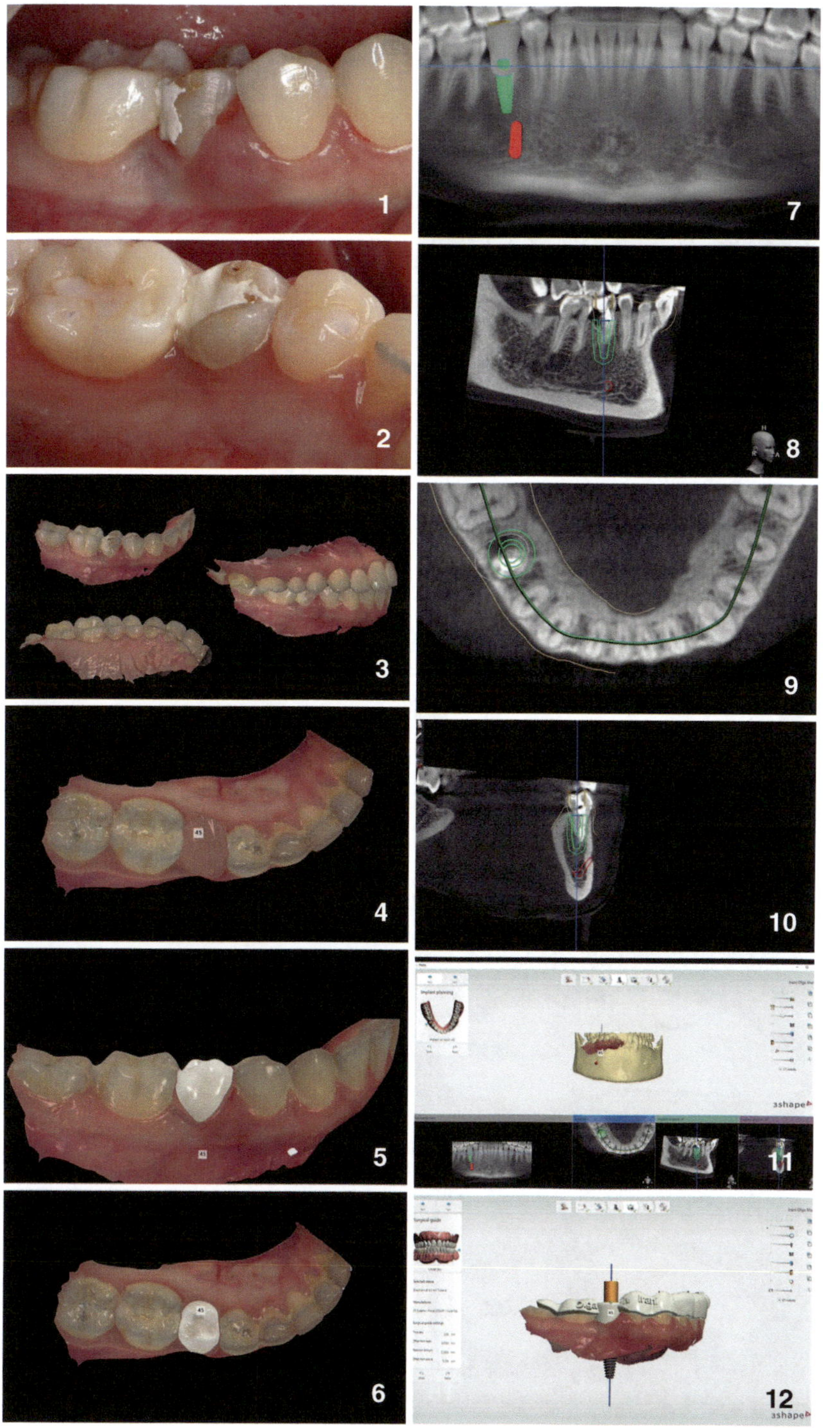
1
7
2
8
3
9
4
10
5
3shape
11
6
12
3shape

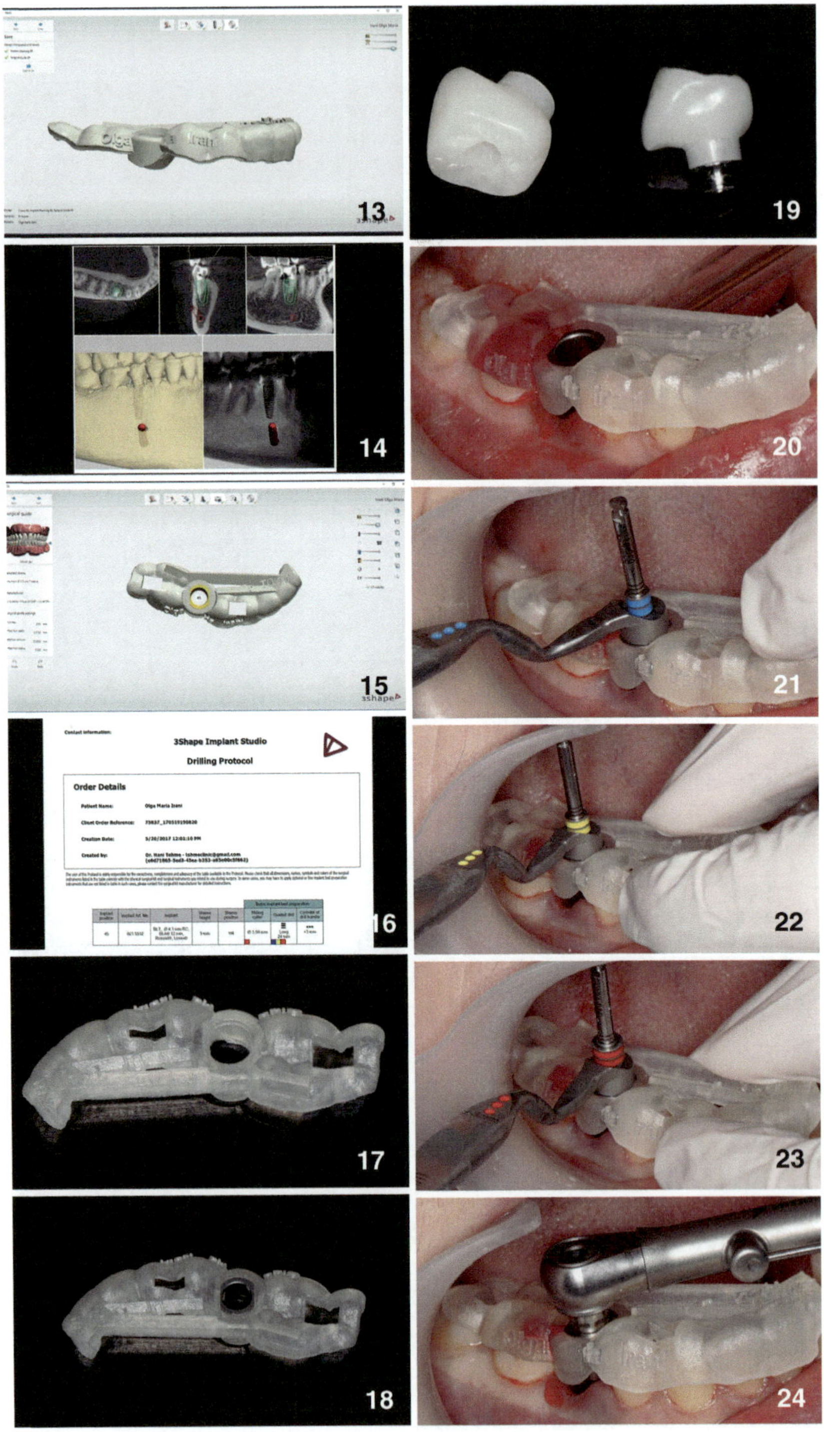

Fig. 7 (continued)

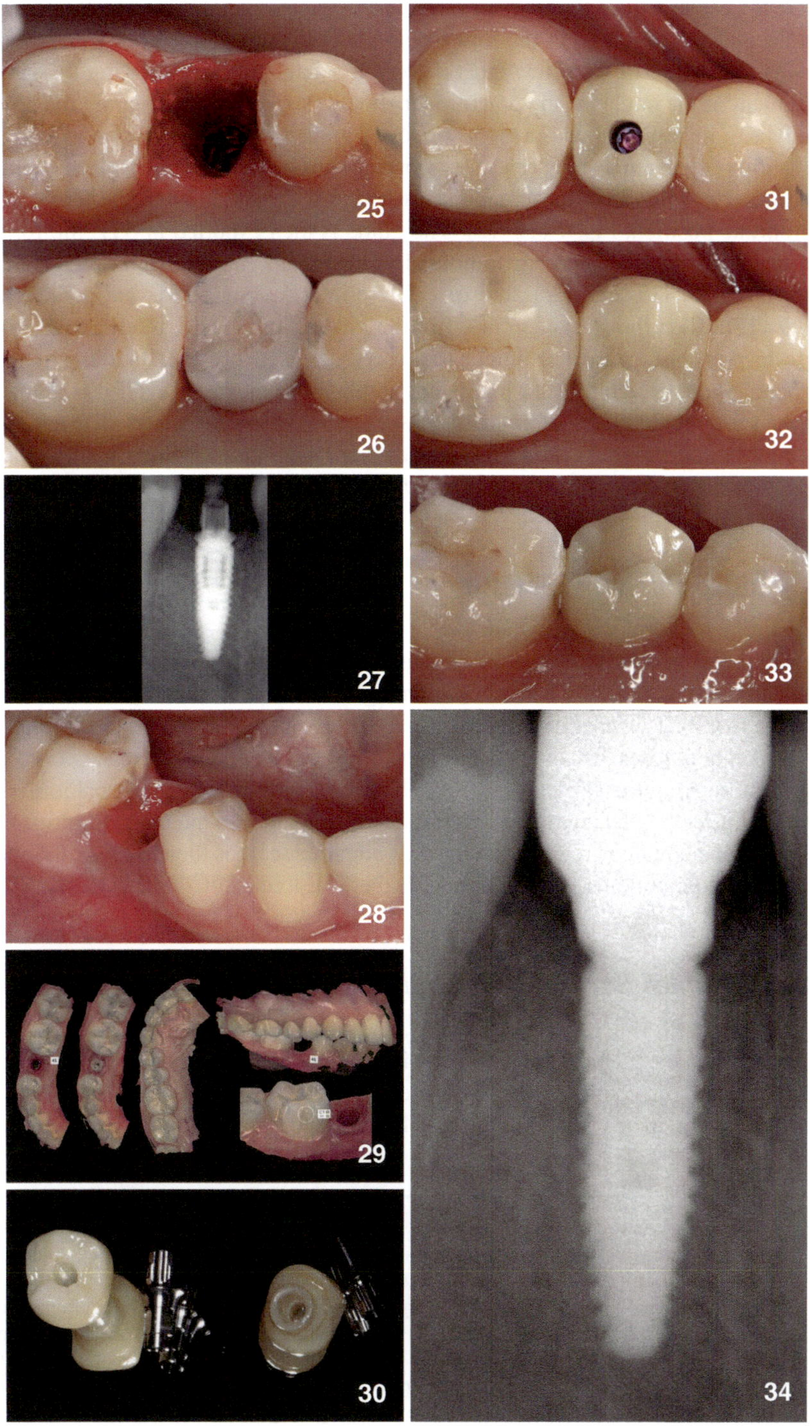

Fig. 7 (continued)

where the center axis of the implant should be in the middle of the premolar which is the place of the axis hole in the future (Fig. 7 (7–11)). When dealing with anterior crowns, the access of the screw must be on the palatal region. Following the virtual placement of the implants, the practitioner should proceed with designing the guide. The type of guide designed is a tooth supported guide with additional bars to increase the rigidity of the guide and prevent its working. It is also advisable to place occlusal windows that will allow the surgeon see whether the guide is fitting perfectly in its appropriate position, Fig. 7 (12–15). The guide is then exported in STL file format with the drilling protocol along with the designed temporary crown, Fig. 7 (16–19). After that, the STL file is printed on a 3D printer, polymerized, and disinfected, Fig. 7 (17). Then the sleeve is placed in the guide, Fig. 7 (18). Tooth extraction is performed in least invasive technique to preserve the bone present. Breaking the buccal bundle bone would prevent immediate implant placement. Even if it is a guided surgery, the prerequisites of immediate surgery must be respected. The guide is placed intraorally and checked for fitting through the windows. Subsequently, drilling begins following the protocol formed by the software, Fig. 7 (20–26).

7 Guided Partially Edentulous Cases

Partially edentulous cases are usually more complicated than the single tooth implant especially if the edentulous area is big enough. It is often found difficult to merge STL file to CBCT when the edentulous space is big or when there are distal free end saddles on both sides. This is because there will not be enough reference points for alignment making the software align the STL file in a wrong spatial position. This can be adjusted by placing two orthodontic mini-implants on the most posterior side of the distal edentulous regions before the patient undergoes the CBCT or the scan. This will the practitioner in superimposing the STL to the DICOM file easily.

Case 2: Guided Surgery in Partially Edentulous Cases

Following is a case of a guided surgery in partially edentulous cases. This guide is a combined guide since it is both tissue and tooth supported. In other words the surgeon did not open a flap since enough keratinized tissues existed, Fig. 8 (1–22).

Fig. 8 (1) Occlusal view of the partially edentulous region. (2) STL file of the patient's upper arch. (3) Placing indications on the software. (4) Designing the suspected future crowns to place the implant guaranteeing a good esthetic result. (5) Cropping patient's CBCT. (6) Locating the panoramic curve horizontal level. (7) Superimposing DICOM and STL files through toggling similar points between both scans. (8) Merged files. (9) Positioning the implants taking the crown designs as a reference. (10 and 11) Surgical guide design and STL file. (12) Drilling protocol. (13) Printed surgical guide without sleeves. (14) Printed surgical guide with sleeves. (15) Frontal view of the surgical guide intraorally. (16) Occlusal view of the surgical guide. (17) Punched tissues. (18) Drilling sequence following the protocol. (19) Occlusal view of implant position. (20) Frontal view of implant position. (21) Healing abutments placed on top of the implants. (22) Periapical X-ray post-guided surgery (With Permission from Dr. Hani Tohme)

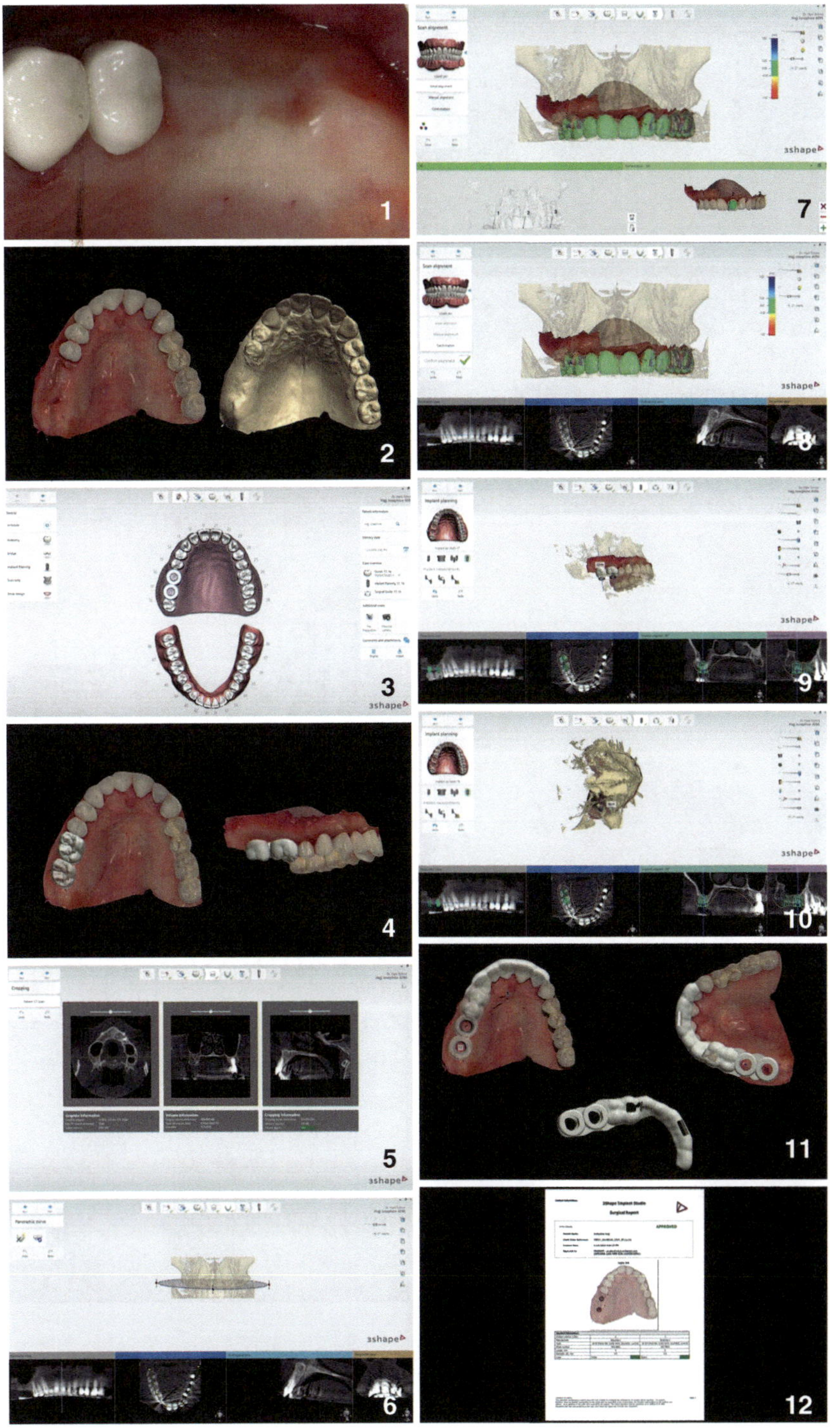
1
2
3
4
5
6
7
8
9
10
11
12

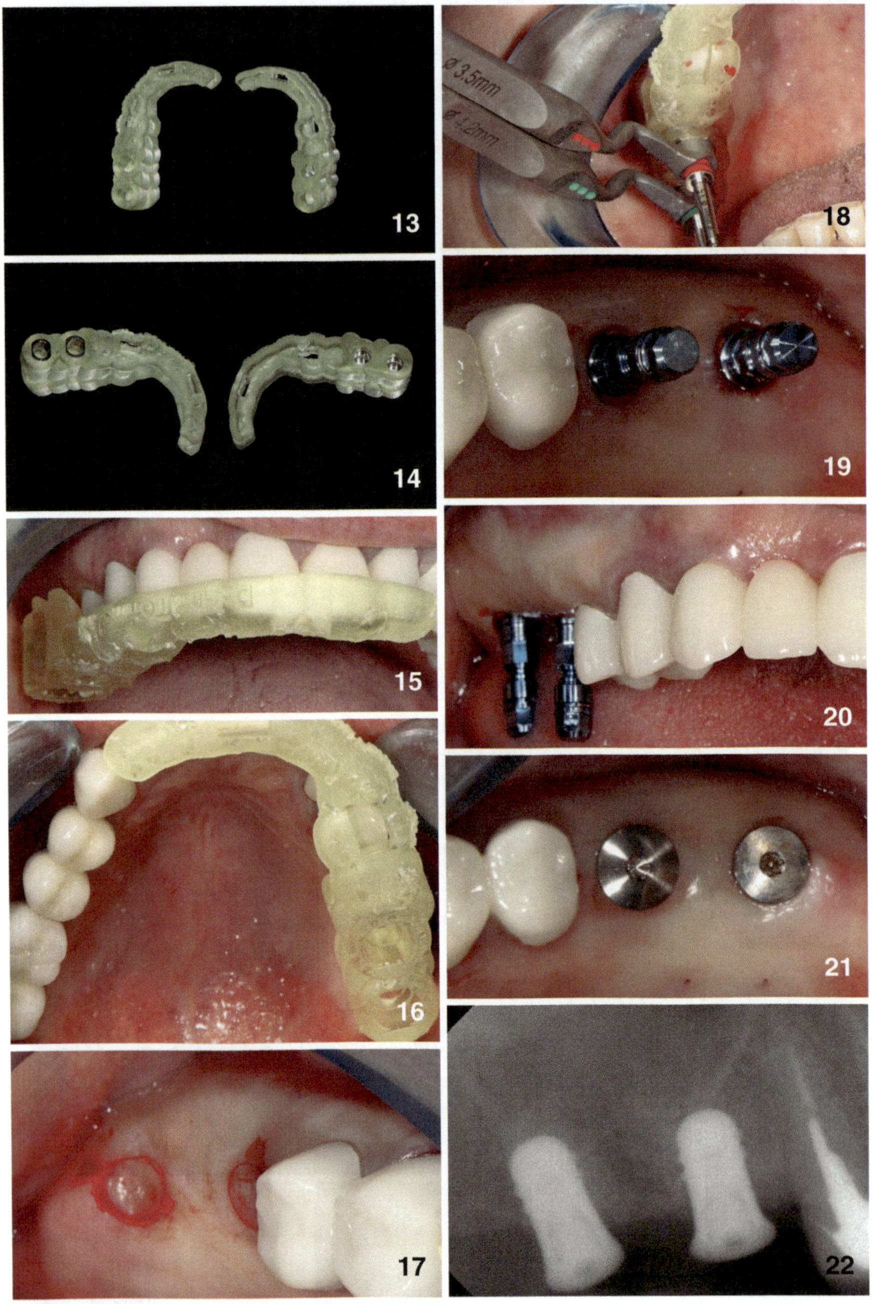

Fig. 8 (continued)

8 Guided Fully Edentulous Cases

Guided full edentulous cases are performed using the double scan protocol (Fig. 9) (1–31). This protocol is mainly composed of scanning the patient first while wearing the denture/radiographic guide with radiopaque markers and scanning the denture alone. The denture should be placed on a foam to make the intaglio surface of the denture clear in the CBCT. The intaglio is necessary because it will be the surface area contacting the soft tissues while performing the guided surgery.

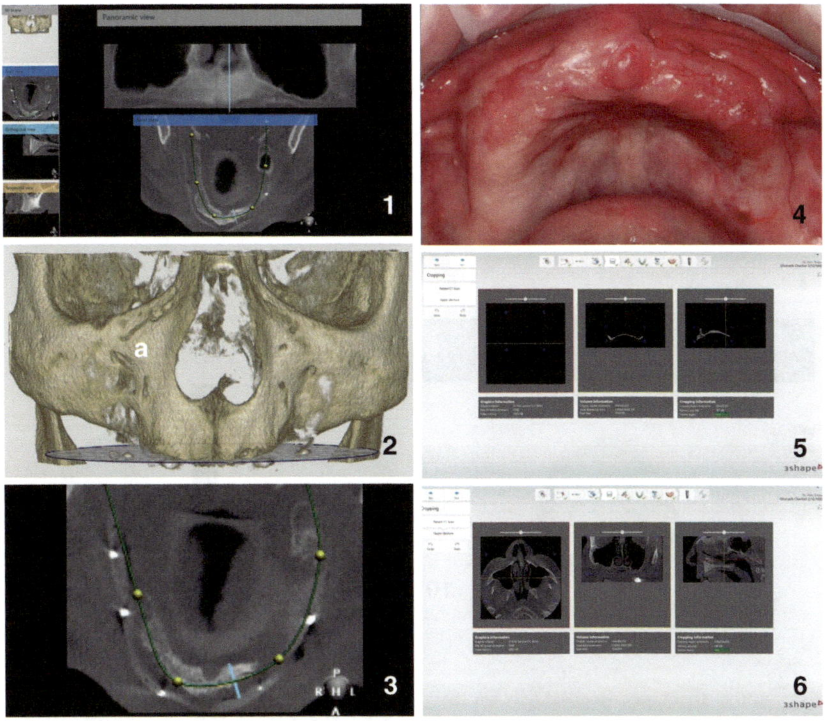

Fig. 9 (1 and 2) Different view of patient's CBCT. (3) Panoramic curve. (4) Edentulous upper arch. (5) Cropping the denture CBCT. (6) Cropping CBCT of patient's jaw with the denture. (7) Denture CBCT. (8) Matching the radio-opaque markers. (9) Denture CBCT superimposed over the patient's CBCT. (10) Marking the intaglio surface. (11) Placing fixation pins. (12) Choosing the implant size and diameter. (13–15) Guide design (notice the added bars to increase rigidity). (16 and 17) Drilling protocol and surgical report. (18) Occlusal view of the maxillary edentulous arch. (19) Guide stabilization intraorally. (20) Punched tissue. (21) Removal of the punched tissues. (22) Performing the guided surgery. (23) Occlusal view of the placed implants. (24) Perforated denture. (25) Screwed temporary abutments. (26) Temporary provisional checked for insertion after screwing temporary abutments on top of implants. (27) Occlusal view of the temporary prosthesis relines intraorally. (28) Intaglio surface of the relined acrylic denture. (29) Frontal view of the denture that was relined and transformed into a fixed bridge acting as a temporary prosthesis. (30) Planned implant position on the software. (31) CBCT of the implants after the guided surgical procedure to check if it was accurate to the planning. (With Permission from Dr. Hani Tohme)

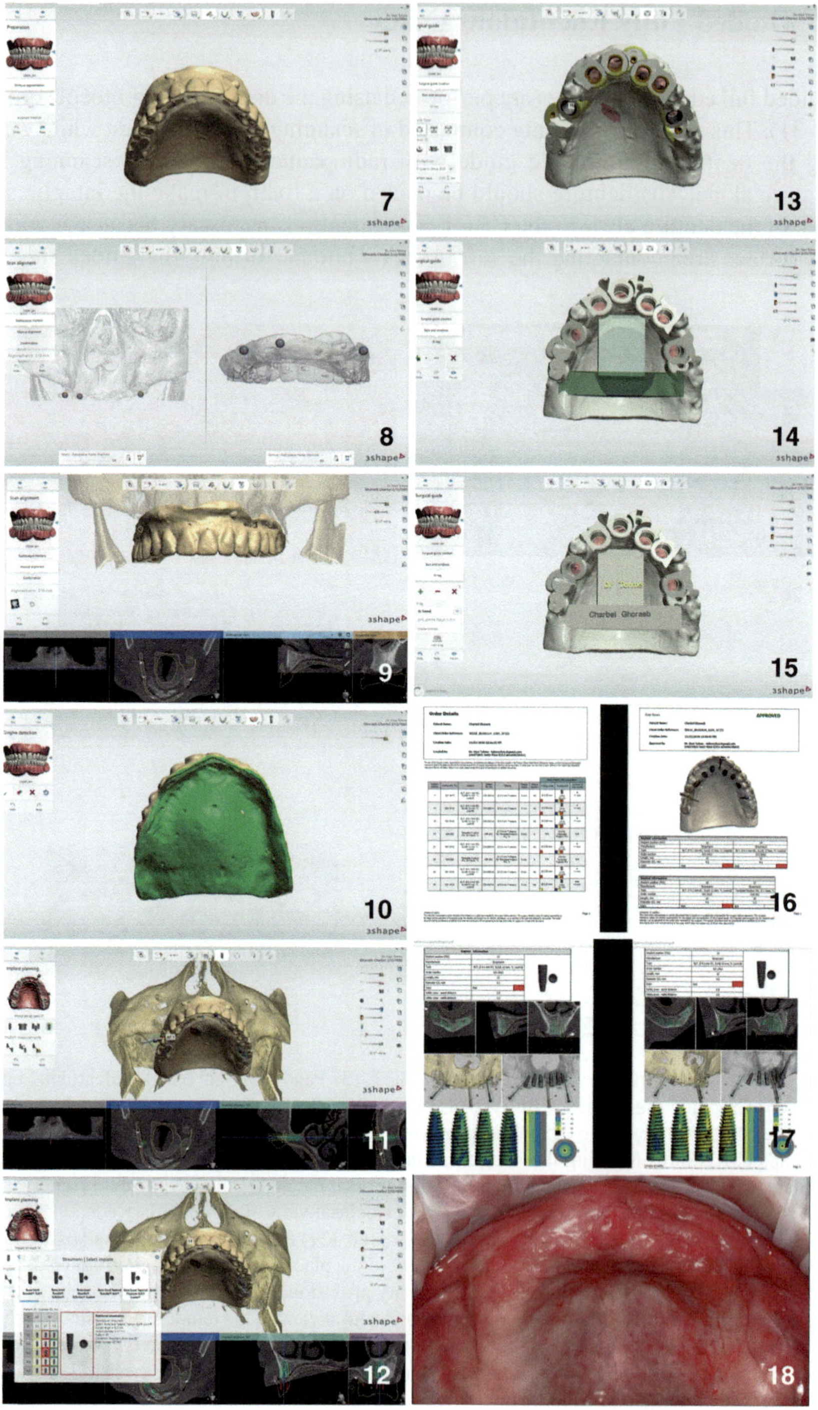

Fig. 9 (continued)

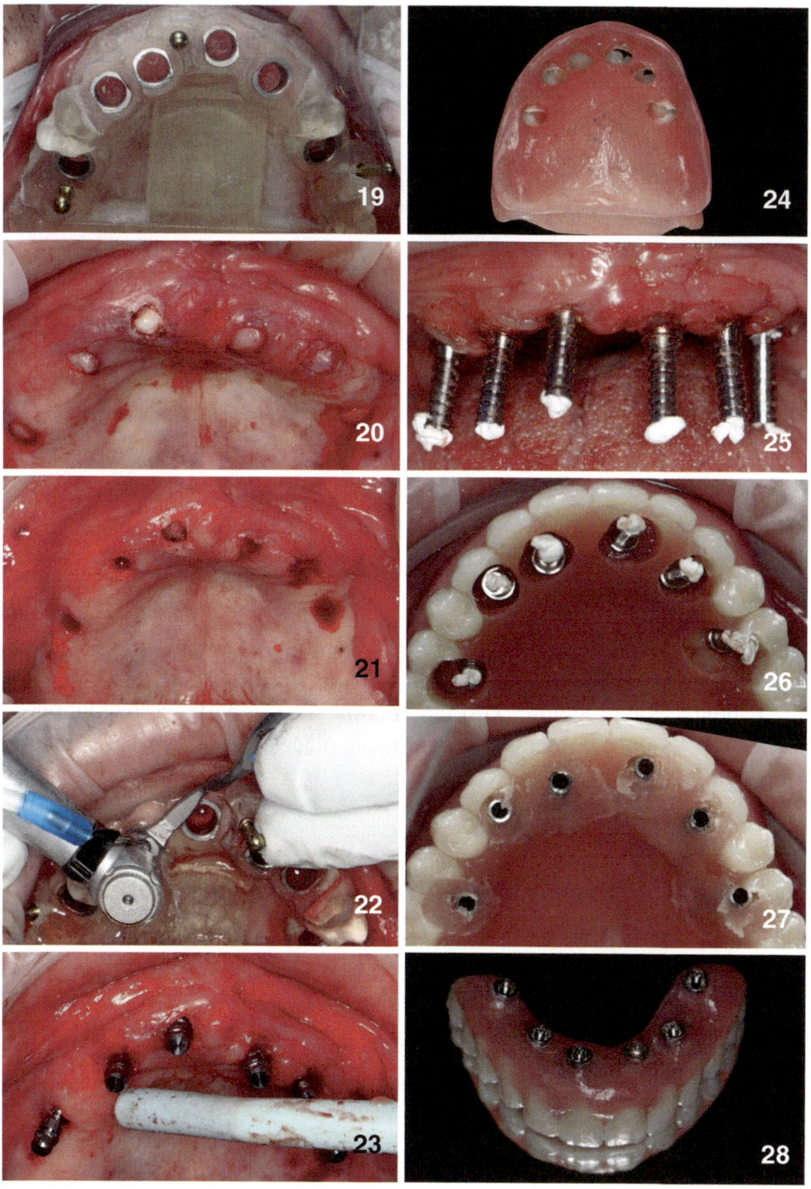

Fig. 9 (continued)

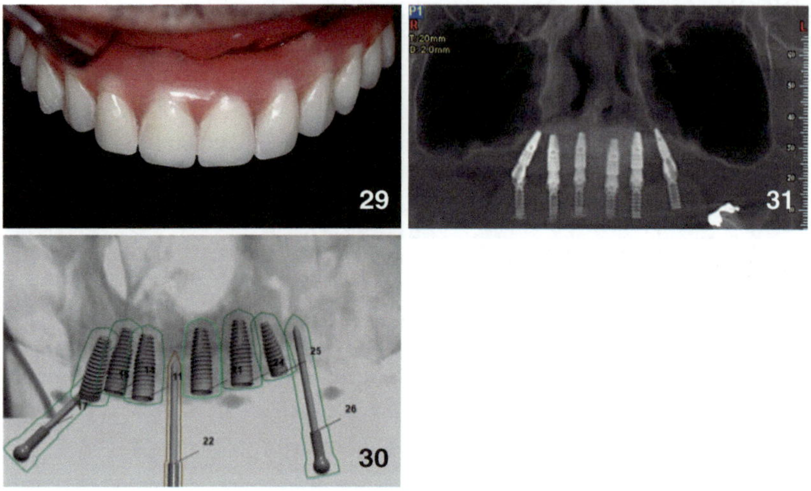

Fig. 9 (continued)

The purpose of performing these two scans is superimposing the two DICOM files over each other using the radiographic markers as a reference resulting in a model of the patient's bone together with the denture. The importance of scanning the denture too is to place implants in the strategic places with a prosthetically driven concept [90, 91].

Case 3: Guided Surgery of a Maxillary Edentulous Case

This case demonstrates the step-by-step workflow of a double or dual scan protocol of an all-on-6 case.

9 Conclusion

Virtual implant planning and guided surgery is attaining recognition and has been suggested to be the benchmark in many complicated dental implant cases. As this advancement is embraced by different implant specialties, there is a related learning curve for each of the program used as well as the procedure performed. This chapter has detailed different software tools that assist implant therapy planning in clinical practice and has also underlined the need to ripen a strict planning protocol that results in successful outcomes. Similarly, accuracy errors can be kept to minimal levels when sources of error are kept in mind during the planning of a case.

References

1. Ganz SD. Computer-aided design/computer-aided manufacturing applications using CT and cone beam CT scanning technology. Dent Clin N Am. 2008;52:777–808.
2. Guerrero ME, Noriega J, Jacobs R. Preoperative implant planning considering alveolar bone GRAFTING needs and complication prediction USING panoramic versus CBCT IMAGES. Imaging Sci Dent. 2014;44:213.
3. Peretz B, Gotler M, Kaffe I. Common errors in digital panoramic radiographs of patients with mixed dentition and patients with permanent dentition. Int J Dent. 2012;2012:1–7.
4. Kumar M, Shanavas M, Sidappa A, Kiran M. Cone beam computed tomography - know its secrets. J Int Oral Health. 2015;7:64–8.
5. Ardekian L, Dodson TB. Complications associated with the placement of dental implants. Oral Maxillofac Surg Clin North Am. 2003;15:243–9.
6. Greenstein G, Cavallaro J, Romanos G, et al. Clinical recommendations for avoiding and managing surgical complications associated with implant dentistry: a review. J Periodontol. 2008;79:1317–29.
7. Ganz SD. Presurgical planning with CT-derived fabrication of surgical guides. J Oral Maxillofac Surg. 2005;63:59–71.
8. Katsoulis J, Enkling N, Takeichi T, et al. Relative bone width of the edentulous maxillary ridge. Clinical implications of digital assessment in presurgical implant planning. Clin Implant Dent Relat Res. 2012;14:213–23.
9. Arisan V, Bolukbasi N, Oksuz L. Computer-assisted flapless implant placement reduces the incidence of surgery-related bacteremia. Clin Oral Investig. 2012;17:1985–93.
10. Sicilia A, Botticelli D. Computer-guided implant therapy and soft- and hard-tissue aspects. The third EAO consensus conference 2012. Clin Oral Implants Res. 2012;23:157–6.
11. Pyo SW, Lim YJ, Koo KT, Lee J. Methods used to assess the 3D accuracy of dental implant positions in computer-guided implant placement: a review. J Clin Med. 2019;8:54.
12. Arisan V, Karabuda CZ, Ozdemir T. Implant surgery using bone- and mucosa-supported stereolithographic guides in totally edentulous jaws: surgical and post-operative outcomes of computer-aided vs. standard techniques. Clin Oral Implants Res. 2010;21:980–8.
13. Farley NE, Kennedy K, McGlumphy EA, Clelland NL. Split-mouth comparison of the accuracy of computer-generated and conventional surgical guides. Int J Oral Maxillofac Implants. 2013;28:563–72.
14. Amorfini L, Migliorati M, Drago S, Silvestrini-Biavati A. Immediately loaded implants in rehabilitation of the maxilla: a two-year randomized clinical trial of guided surgery versus standard procedure. Clin Implant Dent Relat Res. 2017;19:280–95.
15. Vercruyssen M, Laleman I, Jacobs R, Quirynen M. Computer-supported implant planning and guided surgery: a narrative review. Clin Oral Implants Res. 2015;26:69–76.
16. Deeb JG, Bencharit S, Loschiavo CA, Yeung M, Laskin D, Deeb GR. Do implant surgical guides allow an adequate zone of keratinized tissue for flapless surgery? J Oral Maxillofac Surg. 2018;76:2540–50.
17. Sclar AG. Guidelines for flapless surgery. J Oral Maxillofac Surg. 2007;65:20–32.
18. Mijiritsky E, Ben Zaken H, Shacham M, Cinar IC, Tore C, Nagy K, Ganz SD. Variety of surgical guides and protocols for bone reduction prior to implant placement: a narrative review. Int J Environ Res Public Health. 2021;18:2341.
19. Arisan V, Bolukbasi N, Oksuz L. Computer-assisted flapless implant placement reduces the incidence of surgery-related bacteremia. Clin Oral Investig. 2013;17:1985–93.
20. Vercruyssen M, De Laat A, Coucke W, Quirynen M. An RCT comparing patient-centred outcome variables of guided surgery (bone or mucosa supported) with conventional implant placement. J Clin Periodontol. 2014;41:724–32.
21. Pozzi A, Tallarico M, Marchetti M, Scarfo B, Esposito M. Computer-guided versus free-hand placement of immediately loaded dental implants: 1-year post-loading results of a multicentre randomised controlled trial. Eur J Oral Implantol. 2014;7:229–42.

22. Raico Gallardo YN, da Silva-Olivio IRT, Mukai E, Morimoto S, Sesma N, Cordaro L. Accuracy comparison of guided surgery for dental implants according to the tissue of support: a systematic review and meta-analysis. Clin Oral Implants Res. 2017;28:602–12.
23. Boa K, Barrak I, Varga E Jr, Joob-Fancsaly A, Varga E, Piffko J. Intraosseous generation of heat during guided surgical drilling: an ex vivo study of the effect of the temperature of the irrigating fluid. Br J Oral Maxillofac Surg. 2016;54:904–8.
24. Liu YF, Wu JL, Zhang JX, Peng W, Liao WQ. Numerical and experimental analyses on the temperature distribution in the dental implant preparation area when using a surgical guide. J Prosthodont. 2018;27:42–51.
25. Kuhl S, Zurcher S, Mahid T, Muller-Gerbl M, Filippi A, Cattin P. Accuracy of full guided vs. half-guided implant surgery. Clin Oral Implants Res. 2013;24:763–9.
26. Vercruyssen M, Coucke W, Naert I, Jacobs R, Teughels W, Quirynen M. Depth and lateral deviations in guided implant surgery: an RCT comparing guided surgery with mental navigation or the use of a pilot-drill template. Clin Oral Implants Res. 2015;26:1315–20.
27. Younes F, Cosyn J, De Bruyckere T, Cleymaet R, Bouckaert E, Eghbali A. A randomized controlled study on the accuracy of free-handed, pilot-drill guided and fully guided implant surgery in partially edentulous patients. J Clin Periodontol. 2018;45(6):721–32.
28. Arisan V, Karabuda CZ, Mumcu E, Ozdemir T. Implant positioning errors in freehand and computer-aided placement methods: a single-blind clinical comparative study. Int J Oral Maxillofac Implants. 2013;28:190–204.
29. Block MS, Emery RW. Static or dynamic navigation for implant placement-choosing the method of guidance. J Oral Maxillofac Surg. 2016;74:269–77.
30. Jung RE, Schneider D, Ganeles J, Wismeijer D, Zwahlen M, Hämmerle CH, et al. Computer technology applications in surgical implant dentistry: a systematic review. Int J Oral Maxillofac Implants. 2009;24:92–109.
31. Kaewsiri D, Panmekiate S, Subbalekha K, Mattheos N, Pimkhaokham A. The accuracy of static vs. dynamic computer-assisted implant surgery in single tooth space: a randomized controlled trial. Clin Oral Implants Res. 2019;30:505–14.
32. Brief J, Edinger D, Hassfeld S, Eggers G. Accuracy of image-guided implantology. Clin Oral Implants Res. 2005;16:495–501.
33. Block MS, Emery RW, Cullum DR, Sheikh A. Implant placement is more accurate using dynamic navigation. J Oral Maxillofac Surg. 2017;75:1377–86.
34. Sun T-M, Lee H-E, Lan T-H. Comparing accuracy of implant installation with a navigation system (NS), a laboratory guide (LG), NS with LG, and freehand drilling. Int J Environ Res Public Health. 2020;17:2107.
35. Kalaivani G, Balaji VR, Manikandan D, Rohini G. Expectation and reality of guided implant surgery protocol using computer-assisted static and dynamic navigation system at present scenario: evidence-based literature review. J Indian Soc Periodontol. 2020;24:398.
36. Jacobs R, Salmon B, Codari M, Hassan B, Bornstein MM. Cone beam computed tomography in implant dentistry: recommendations for clinical use. BMC Oral Health. 2018;15(18):88.
37. Dreiseidler T, Tandon D, Kreppel M, Neugebauer J, Mischkowski RA, Zinser MJ, Zöller JE. CBCT device dependency on the transfer accuracy from computer-aided implantology procedures. Clin Oral Implants Res. 2012;23:1089–97.
38. Tyndall DA, Price JB, Tetradis S, Ganz SD, Hildebolt C, Scarfe WC. American Academy of Oral and maxillofacial radiology. Position statement of the American Academy of Oral and maxillofacial radiology on selection criteria for the use of radiology in dental implantology with emphasis on cone beam computed tomography. Oral Surg Oral Med Oral Pathol Oral Radiol. 2012;113:817–26.
39. Chmielewski K, Chmielewska M. Guided surgery. Dental print 3D; 2020.
40. Tahmaseb A, Wismeijer D, Coucke W, Derksen W. Computer technology applications in surgical implant dentistry: a systematic review. Int J Oral Maxillofac Implants. 2014;29 Suppl:25–42.

41. Nagata K, Fuchigami K, Hoshi N, Atsumi M, Kimoto K, Kawana H. Accuracy of guided surgery using the silicon impression and digital impression method for the mandibular free end: a comparative study. Int J Implant Dent. 2021;12(7):2.
42. Mora MA, Chenin DL, Arce RM. Software tools and surgical guides in dental-implant-guided surgery. Dent Clin N Am. 2014;58:597–626.
43. Mattera M, Reginelli A, Bartollino S, Russo C, Barile A, Albano D, Mauri G, Messina C, Cappabianca S, Guglielmi G. Imaging of metabolic bone disease. Acta Biomed. 2018;89:197–207.
44. Cavallaro J, Tsuji S, Chiu TS, Greenstein G. Management of the nasopalatine canal and foramen associated with dental implant therapy. Compend Contin Educ Dent. 2016;38:367–72.
45. Borgonovo A, Fabbri A, Boninsegna R, Dolci M, Censi. Displacement of a dental implant into the maxillary sinus: case series. Minerva Stomatol. 2010;59:45–54.
46. Neiva RF, Gapski R, Wang HL. Morphometric analysis of implant-related anatomy in Caucasian skulls. J Periodontol. 2004;75:1061–7.
47. Longoni S, Sartori M, Braun M, et al. Lingual vascular canals of the mandible: the risk of bleeding complications during implant procedures. Implant Dent. 2007;16:131–8.
48. Kilic E, Doganay S, Ulu M, et al. Determination of lingual vascular canals in the interforaminal region before implant surgery to prevent life-threatening bleeding complications. Clin Oral Implants Res. 2012;25:90–3.
49. Juodzbalys G, Wang HL, Sabalys G. Injury of the inferior alveolar nerve during implant placement: a literature review. J Oral Maxillofac Res. 2011;2(1):e1.
50. Klinge B, Petersson A, Maly P. Location of the mandibular canal: comparison of macroscopic findings, conventional radiography, and computed tomography. Int J Oral Maxillofac Implants. 1989;4:327–32.
51. Tarnow DP, Magner AW, Fletcher P. The effect of the distance from the contact point to the crest of bone on the presence or absence of the interproximal dental papilla. J Periodontol. 1992;63:995–6.
52. Tarnow DP, Cho SC, Wallace SS. The effect of inter-implant distance on the height of inter-implant bone crest. J Periodontol. 2000;71:546–9.
53. Spray JR, Black CG, Morris HF, et al. The influence of bone thickness on facial marginal bone response: stage 1 placement through stage 2 uncovering. Ann Periodontol. 2000;5:119–28.
54. Buser D, Martin W, Belser UC. Optimizing esthetics for implant restorations in the anterior maxilla: anatomic and surgical considerations. Int J Oral Maxillofac Implants. 2004; 19:43–61.
55. Marlière DAA, Demètrio MS, Picinini LS, Oliveira RG, Netto HDMC. Accuracy of computer-guided surgery for dental implant placement in fully edentulous patients: a systematic review. Eur J Dent. 2018;12:153–60.
56. Tagger Green N, Machtei EE, Horwitz J, et al. Fracture of dental implants: literature review and report of a case. Implant Dent. 2002;11:137–43.
57. Kessler A, Hickel R, Reymus M. 3D printing in dentistry-state of the art. Oper Dent. 2020;45:30–40.
58. Kim SY, Shin YS, Jung HD, Hwang CJ, Baik HS, Cha JY. Precision and trueness of dental models manufactured with different 3-dimensional printing techniques. Am J Orthod Dentofac Orthop. 2018;153:144–53.
59. Oberoi G, Nitsch S, Edelmayer M, Janjić K, Müller AS, Agis H. 3D printing—encompassing the facets of dentistry. Front Bioeng Biotechnol. 2018;6:172.
60. Rungrojwittayakul O, Kan JY, Shiozaki K, Swamidass RS, Goodacre BJ, Goodacre CJ, Lozada JL. Accuracy of 3D printed models created by two Technologies of Printers with different designs of Model Base. J Prosthodont. 2020;29:124–8.
61. Brown GB, Currier GF, Kadioglu O, Kierl JP. Accuracy of 3-dimensional printed dental models reconstructed from digital intraoral impressions. Am J Orthod Dentofac Orthop. 2018;154:733–9.

62. Favero CS, English JD, Cozad BE, Wirthlin JO, Short MM, Kasper FK. Effect of print layer height and printer type on the accuracy of 3-dimensional printed orthodontic models. Am J Orthod Dentofac Orthop. 2017;152:557–65.
63. Park M-E, Shin S-Y. Three-dimensional comparative study on the accuracy and reproducibility of dental casts fabricated by 3D printers. J Prosthet Dent. 2018;119:861.
64. Sun Y, Ding Q, Tang L, Zhang L, Sun Y, Xie Q. Accuracy of a chairside fused deposition modeling 3D-printed single-tooth surgical template for implant placement: an in vitro comparison with a light cured template. J Cranio-Maxillofac Surg. 2019;47:1216–21.
65. Di Giacomo GA, Cury PR, de Araujo NS, Sendyk WR, Sendyk CL. Clinical application of stereolithographic surgical guides for implant placement: preliminary results. J Periodontol. 2005;76:503–7.
66. Anunmana C, Ueawitthayasuporn C, Kiattavorncharoen S, Thanasrisuebwong P. In vitro comparison of surgical implant placement accuracy using guides fabricated by three different additive technologies. Appl Sci. 2020;10:7791.
67. Smith PN, Palenik CJ, Blanchard SB. Microbial contamination and the sterilization/disinfection of surgical guides used in the placement of endosteal implants. Int J Oral Maxillofac Implants. 2011;26:274–81.
68. Colombo M, et al. Clinical applications and effectiveness of guided implant surgery: a critical review based on randomized controlled trials. BMC Oral Health. 2016;13(2017):150.
69. Moon SY, Lee KR, Kim SG, Son MK. Clinical problems of computer-guided implant surgery. Maxillofac Plast Reconstr Surg. 2016;38:15.
70. Cassetta M, Bellardini M. How much does experience in guided implant surgery play a role in accuracy? A randomized controlled pilot study. Int J Oral Maxillofac Surg. 2017;46:922–30.
71. Cassetta M, Altieri F, Giansanti M, Bellardini M, Brandetti G, Piccoli L. Is there a learning curve in static computer-assisted implant surgery? A prospective clinical study. Int J Oral Maxillofac Surg. 2020;49:1335–42. https://doi.org/10.1016/j.ijom.2020.03.007; Epub 2020 Mar 23
72. Jones A. Accuracy of mucosa supported guided dental implant surgery. Clin Case Reports. 2018;6:2131–9.
73. Sannino G, Gherlone EF. Thermal changes during guided flapless implant site preparation: a comparative study. Int J Oral Maxillofac Implants. 2018;33(3):671–7.
74. Dreiseidler T, Tandon D, Kreppel M, Neugebauer J, Mischkowski RA, Zinser MJ, et al. CBCT device dependency on the transfer accuracy from computer-guided implantology procedures. Clin Oral Implants Res. 2012;23:1089–97.
75. Hassan B, Couto Souza P, Jacobs R, de Azambuja Berti S, van der Stelt P. Influence of scanning and reconstruction parameters on quality of three-dimensional surface models of the dental arches from cone beam computed tomography. Clin Oral Investig. 2010;14:303–10.
76. Spin-Neto R, Gotfredsen E, Wenzel A. Impact of voxel size variation on CBCT-based diagnostic outcome in dentistry: a systematic review. J Digit Imaging. 2013;26:813–20.
77. Widmann G, Bale RJ. Accuracy in computer-aided implant surgery--a review. Int J Oral Maxillofac Implants. 2006;21:305–13.
78. Pettersson A, Komiyama A, Hultin M, Näsström K, Klinge B. Accuracy of virtually planned and template guided implant surgery on edentate patients. Clin Implant Dent Relat Res. 2012;14:527–37.
79. Meloni SM, De Riu G, Pisano M, Cattina G, Tullio A. Implant treatment soft- ware planning and guided flapless surgery with immediate. Eur J Oral Implantol. 2020;3:245–51.
80. Holst S, Blatz MB, Eitner S. Precision for computer-guided implant placement: using 3D planning software and fixed intraoral reference points. J Oral Maxillofac Surg. 2007;65:393–9.
81. Viegas VN, Dutra V, Pagnoncelli RM, de Oliveira MG. Transference of virtual planning and planning over biomedical prototypes for dental implant placement using guided surgery. Clin Oral Implants. 2010;21:290–5.

82. Flügge T, Derksen W, Te Poel J, Hassan B, Nelson K, Wismeijer D. Registration of cone beam computed tomography data and intraoral surface scans - a prerequisite for guided implant surgery with CAD/CAM drilling guides. Clin Oral Implants Res. 2017;28:1113–8.
83. Yeung M, Abdulmajeed A, Carrico CK, Deeb GR, Bencharit S. Accuracy and precision of 3D-printed implant surgical guides with different implant systems: an in vitro study. J Prosthet Dent. 2020;12:821–8.
84. Palazzo G, Ronsivalle V, Oteri G, Lo Giudice A, Toro C, Campagna P, Patini R, Bocchieri S, Bianchi A, Isola G. Comparison between additive and subtractive CAD-CAM technique to produce orthognathic surgical splints: a personalized approach. J Pers Med. 2020;10:273.
85. Malo P, de Araujo NM, Lopes A. The use of computer-guided flapless implant surgery and four implants placed in immediate function to support a fixed denture: preliminary results after a mean follow-up period of thirteen months. J Prosthet Dent. 2007;97:S26–34.
86. Yong LT, Moy PK. Complications of computer-guided-design/computer- guided-machining-guided (NobelGuide) surgical implant placement: an evaluation of early clinical results. Clin Implant Dent Relat Res. 2008;10:123–7.
87. Meloni SM, De Riu G, Pisano M, Massarelli O, Tullio A. Computer assisted dental rehabilitation in free flaps reconstructed jaws: one. Br J Oral Maxillofac Surg. 2012;50:726–31.
88. Cassetta M, Di Mambro A, Giansanti M, Stefanelli LV, Cavallini C. The intrinsic error of a stereolithographic surgical template in implant guided surgery. Int J Oral Maxillofac Surg. 2013;42:264–75.
89. Friberg B, Sennerby L, Gröndahl K, Bergström C, Bäck T, Lekholm U. On cutting torque measurements during implant placement: a 3-year clinical prospective study. Clin Implant Dent Relat Res. 1999;1:75–83.
90. Marchack CB, Moy PK. The use of a custom template for immediate loading with the definitive prosthesis: a clinical report. J Calif Dent Assoc. 2003;31:925–9.
91. Lal K, White GS, Morea DN, Wright RF. Use of stereolithographic templates for surgical and prosthodontic implant planning and placement. Part II a clinical report. J Prosthodont. 2006;15:117–22.

Static Surgical Guides and Dynamic Navigation in Implant Surgery

Reihaneh G. Mauer, Aida Shadrav, and Mahmood Dashti

Every successful treatment starts with a comprehensive examination of the patient, and implant treatment planning is not an exception. Implant treatment planning is restoratively driven and must include multiple disciplinary evaluations [1]. In this chapter, we review factors that may affect implant surgery, specifically the implant placement. Furthermore, we will demonstrate how to construct a conventional surgical guide for a single tooth implant in the dental office and the process of creating a digitally planned guide.

Accuracy of implant placement plays an important role in its long-term success. Many studies have shown that mispositioning of implants may jeopardize the final result [2–4].

Implant placement can be executed in two ways: guided surgery or free-hand placement. Although practitioners may choose to place the implants free-hand, the accuracy of the implant placement would rely on factors like the level of expertise and overcoming the limitations of physical oral space [5, 6]. Surgical guides increase the accuracy of implant placement and positively influence the prosthesis success [5].

New technology may play a large role in the patient's acceptance of the treatment plan and the clinician's comfort to proceed with the surgical treatment. The 3D models and digital wax-ups can aid the patient in visualizing the final results. Similarly, the computer-aided technology may aid the clinicians place the implant,

R. G. Mauer (✉)
Periodontist at Mauer Periodontics & Implant Dentistry, LLC, Fort Myers, FL, USA

A. Shadrav
UCLA School of Dentistry, Los Angeles, CA, USA

M. Dashti
Med Spa, Esfahan, Iran

S. A. Parhiz et al. (eds.), *Navigation in Oral and Maxillofacial Surgery*,
https://doi.org/10.1007/978-3-031-06223-0_6

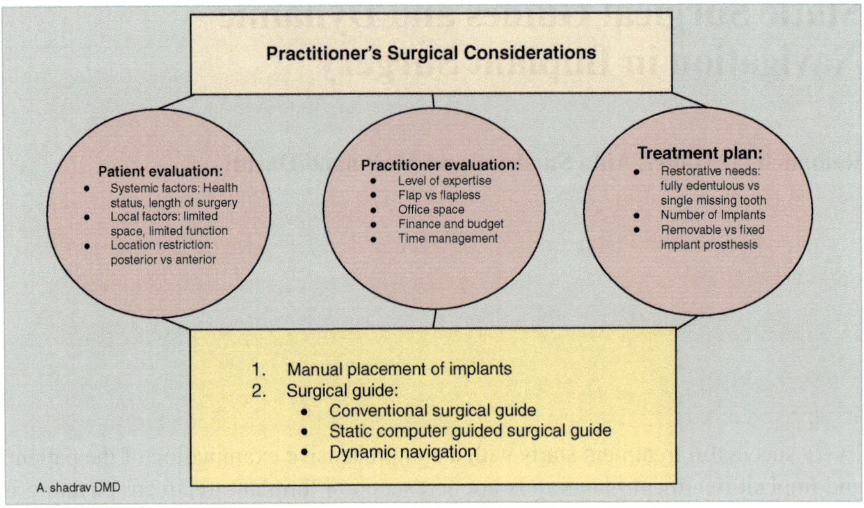

Fig. 1 Factors that may affect the practitioner's decision surgical phase of implant placement

simplify treatment steps including taking impressions thus increasing patient comfort, as well as decreasing surgical complication. It will also help the surgical practitioner to collaborate with a restorative clinician for precise placement [7].

In order to have a successful and accurate guide, all team members including laboratory technician, restorative, and surgical clinicians should pay attention to all the details from the starting point such as clinical evaluation and taking radiographs, to the final surgical step of placing implant through the guide [8].

General surgical guides can be classified into two groups: static and dynamic. Static guides can be fabricated conventionally by traditional impression material or through digital intraoral scanners and computer-guided CAD/CAM. Dynamic navigation is based on computer-guided planned surgeries; therefore, there is no need for a physical surgical guide. The conventional guides can be made in the office or sent to a laboratory. Factors which may affect the practitioner's decisions on implant surgery are presented in Fig. 1.

Multiple studies have compared the deviation of the implant placement [9, 10].

Although the digital planning and computerized surgical guides are reliable, there are some factors that may affect the degree of deviation and accuracy along the process [11].

Table 1 summarizes the parameters that may affect the accuracy of digital plan while taking the cone beam CT.

1 Steps Involved in Implant Placement

There are multiple steps of implant treatment planning prior to performing the surgical phase. The steps are arranged in the following order [11]:

Table 1 Factors affecting the precision and accuracy of the digital image

Cone beam computed tomography (CBCT) machine	1. Voxel box: the smaller the voxel the better the accuracy [12] 2. Patient position and angulation [13] 3. Image artifacts, beam hardening, metal restoration [14]
Patient	1. Patient movement at the time of taking scan 2. Soft tissue thickness [12] 3. Physical size of the jaws [12]
Practitioner	1. Level of expertise [15] 2. Clinical environment [15]

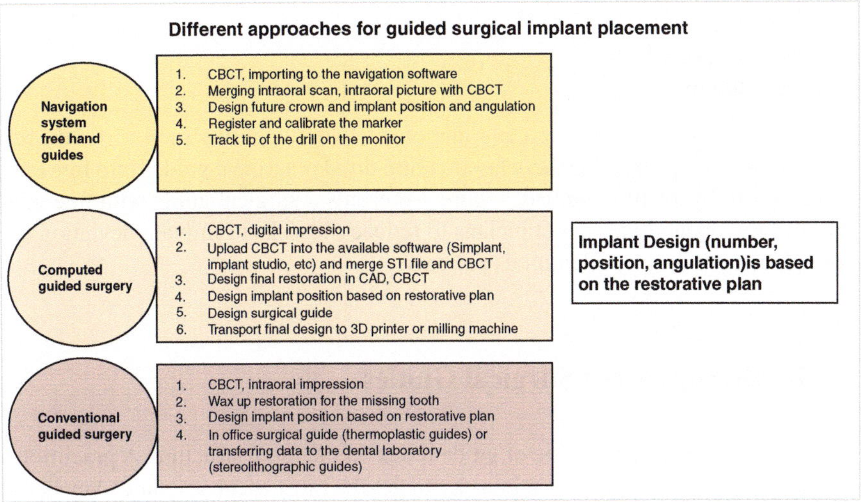

Fig. 2 Three different approaches to surgical implant placement

1. Clinical comprehensive examination (medical records, intra- and extraoral examination).
2. Taking appropriate radiographs and existing digital data (intraoral scans, CBCT, STI files).
3. Implant planning (software virtual plan) and collaborative accountability [7].
4. Computer-aided design and manufacturing of surgical guides (CAD/CAM).
5. Surgical implant placement.

Appropriate digital technology helps the dental practitioners to develop a precise, highly predictive, and suitable treatment based on the patient's needs preoperatively rather than intraoperatively [7].

The different methods for placing implants is depicted in Fig. 2. A clinician may choose the surgical technique based on expertise, finance, number of implants, and patient-based factors.

2 Surgical Guide Classification

In general, a surgical guide is defined as template used by the dental surgeon to place implants with high accuracy, precision, and minimal invasive surgery [16].

A surgical guide should be firm, transparent, stable, autoclavable, easy to use, and adjustable [17]. In addition, the guide should be biocompatible.

All surgical guides have two parts: the first part is the supporting part which fits on the patient's tooth, tissue, and bone and the second part is the drilling guide cylinder that is designed based on available space, implant size, and implant system [5].

Based on the type of support, implant surgical guides are divided into three categories:

1. Tooth supported.
2. Tissue supported.
3. Bone supported.

Surgical guides can be the combination of two categories such as tooth- and tissue-supported guides. Further classification divides surgical guides into free open access, partially, or fully guided. Figure 3 presents a surgical guide with free open access. Free open guides aid clinicians to reduce the risks of implant deviation and miss placement in fully edentulous patients.

3 Tooth-Supported Surgical Guides

As the name suggests, this type of guide relies on the tooth structure. A practitioner should use the latest impression in order to get the most accurate guide. Any deformity can result in difficult adaptation of the guide intraorally. It is very important to

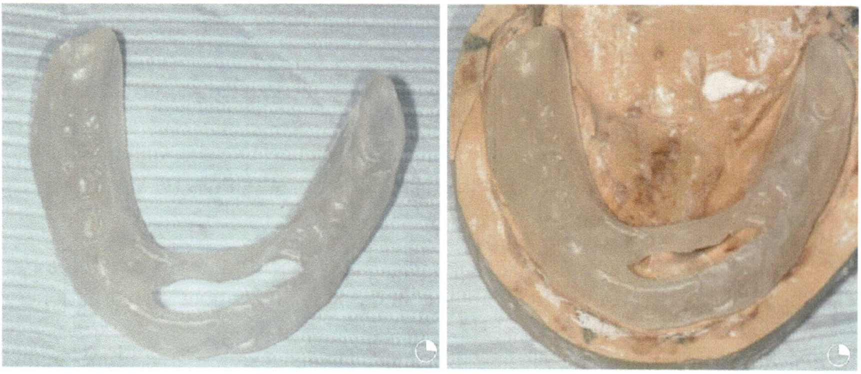

Fig. 3 Free open access surgical guide made in-office for placement of implants #22 and 24

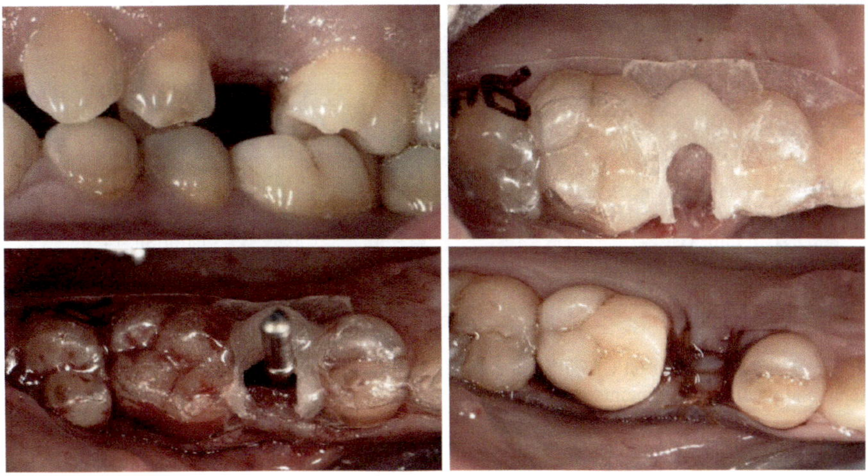

Fig. 4 A tooth-supported conventional surgical guide is demonstrated in the picture. The guide should be checked for accuracy and stability first. The lower left picture demonstrates how the implant screw drive passes through the opening of the guide as it was planned

check the guide accuracy on the cast and in the mouth before proceeding to the surgery [18]. Figure 4 presents an in-office made tooth supported guide for implant #13.

4 Mucosal Tissue-Supported Surgical Guides

This type of the surgical guide will fit on the mucosal tissue and needs to be secured by fixation screws. It is important to check the accuracy of the guide by providing an intraoral surgical index. The guide should accurately fit on the mucosa while the jaw relationships are in centric relations.

5 Bone-Supported Surgical Guides

This type of guide will sit on the bone and should be examined on the digital or stereolithographic bone model before proceeding with the surgery. The clinician should ensure high accuracy of guide location by looking at the teeth and the location of anatomical structures intraorally.

Figures 5, 6 and 7 present a digital bone-supported metal surgical guide made by a dental laboratory. The digital plan is discussed between laboratory and clinician. The printed paper for the day of surgery is shown in Fig. 5. The pictures are courtesy of Viruet Periodontics and Implant Dentistry.

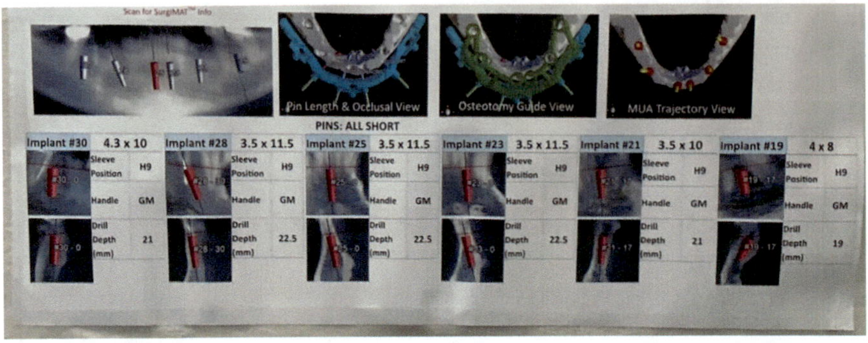

Fig. 5 Digital planning on CBCT for a patient. Treatment plan includes extraction of remaining teeth and placing five implants immediately

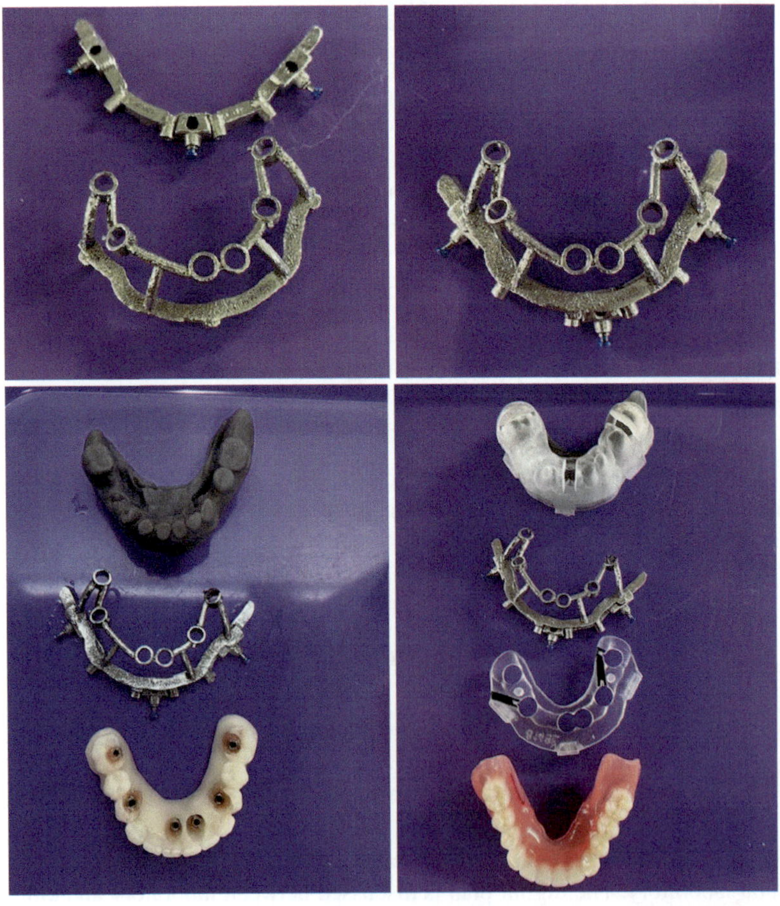

Fig. 6 Two-piece guides, fabricated by a dental laboratory, include bone reduction piece and implant placement guide tubes. The guide is designed for the placement of six implants for a fully edentulous mandible. The restorative plan includes a reconstruction by fixed prosthesis implant restorations. Left picture presents a printed model in gray, metal surgical guide, and an extra temporary printed denture with screw locations. Right picture demonstrates a fitting printed guide on the model, two-piece surgical guide, abutment guide, and temporary denture made by the laboratory

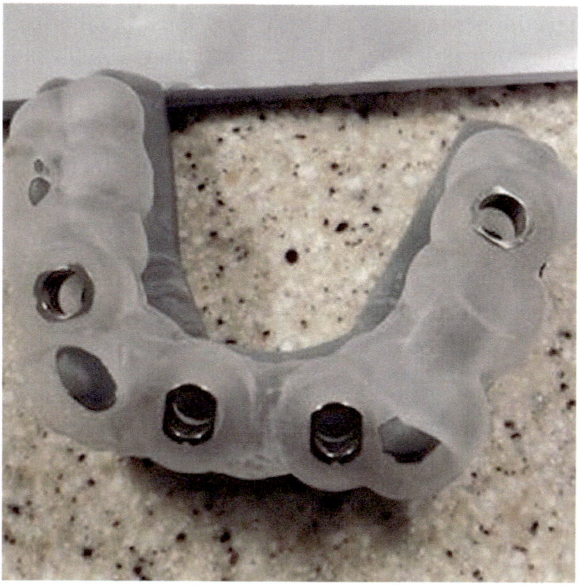

Fig. 7 Fully guided surgical stent with no fixation screws placed on the model of mandible, fabricated by the laboratory. The metal tubes direct the clinician in placement and angulation of the implant

6 Fully Guided Versus Partially Guided Surgical Guides

A fully guided surgical stent includes the base of the guide and tubes that are built in. The fully guided surgical stent allows the clinicians to perform each osteotomy in previously planned size and depth. This signifies that the clinician is restricted in changing the angulation or depth of the drill through the guide. Every implant system has its own surgical kit that matches with the surgical guides, along with the manufacturer's instructions. Figure 7 presents a sample of the fully guided tooth-supported surgical guide. The printed model will be provided to the clinician to ensure the fit and accuracy of the guide.

A partial surgical guide aids the clinician for the pilot drill osteotomy. Further osteotomy preparation and implant placement would be performed with a free-hand technique.

Research comparing fully guided and partially guided implant surgery has shown that fully guided surgical guides are more accurate in implant deviation [19].

7 Steps in Fabricating a Surgical Guide

The comprehensive examination includes the intra- and extraoral, laboratory examination such as primary impressions for making study casts and appropriate radiographs. Implementing CBCT as an adjunctive diagnostic tool has been growing and is recognized as standard of care in dental implant treatment [20]. When a practitioner requests a CBCT, they must familiarize themselves with normal and pathological findings in order to avoid any complications and harm to the patient.

There are three ways to make a surgical guide:

1. Conventional guides made in-office or by laboratory technicians.
2. Computer-aided design/computer-aided manufacture technique (CAD/CAM), printed, and milled [5, 21].
3. CBCT planned dynamic navigation system.

As mentioned previously, surgical guides are classified into two main groups: static surgical guides and dynamic navigation guides.

8 Conventional Single Implant Guide

The steps for making a conventional surgical guide are depicted in Figs. 8, 9, 10, 11, 12, 13 and 14. The clinician must sterilize any surgical guide before placing intraorally. This could be done with cold or heat sterilization methods based on the guide's material.

9 Static Surgical Guides, Stereolithography

Stereolithography prototyping method is used to fabricate surgical guides by a polymerization process with a laser. The surgical guide produced by the prototyping method is a strong, hard 3D copy of human anatomy [22]. It offers benefits such as

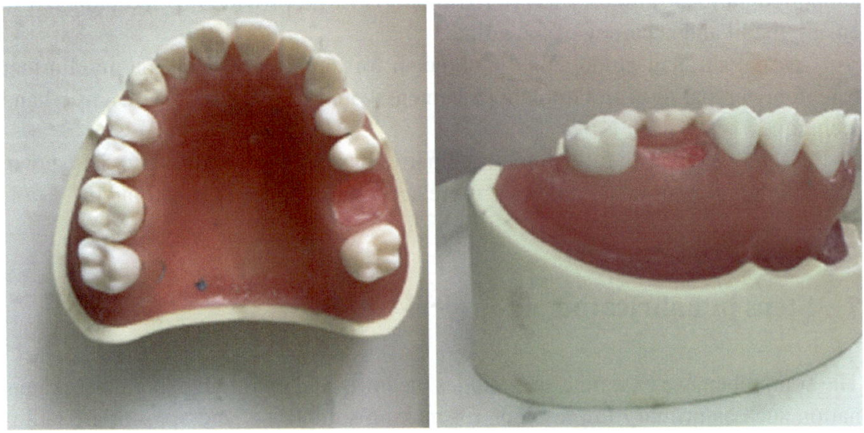

Fig. 8 A typodont is chosen to show the process of making a conventional surgical guide for placing implant #14. Left picture: occlusal view of the initial typodont. Right picture: Buccal view of the initial typodont

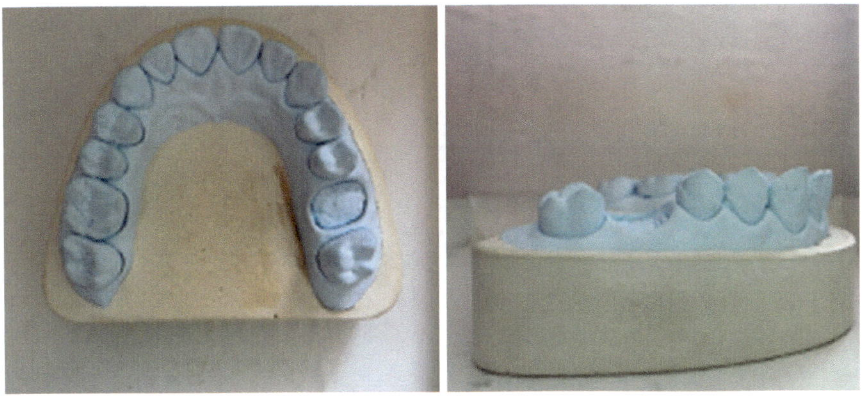

Fig. 9 Left picture: Occlusal view of the gypsum cast. Right picture: Buccal view of the gypsum cast

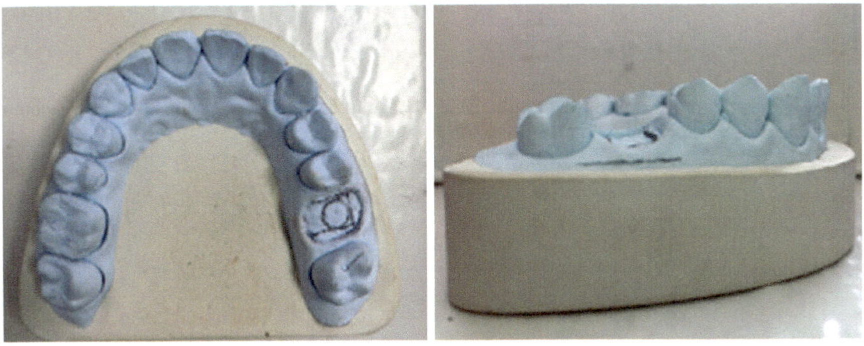

Fig. 10 Left picture: Occlusal view of measurement of implant position on cast. Right picture: Buccal view of measurement of implant position on cast

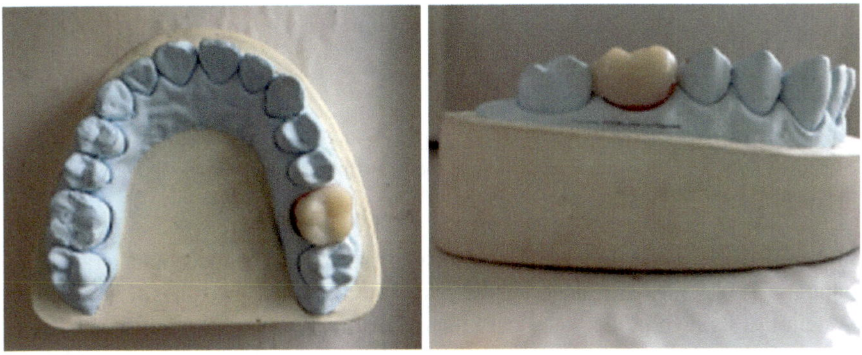

Fig. 11 Left picture: Occlusal view of composite template of implant prosthetic position on cast. Right picture: Buccal view of composite template of implant prosthetic position on cast

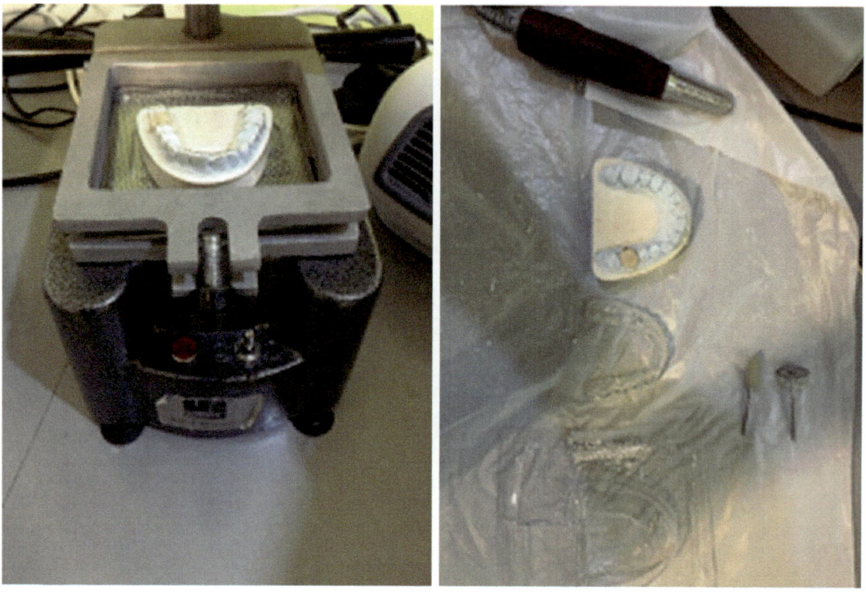

Fig. 12 Left picture: Creating the guide using a 1.5 mm hard template with Ultradent vacuum. Right picture: Cutting, removing, and polishing the guide

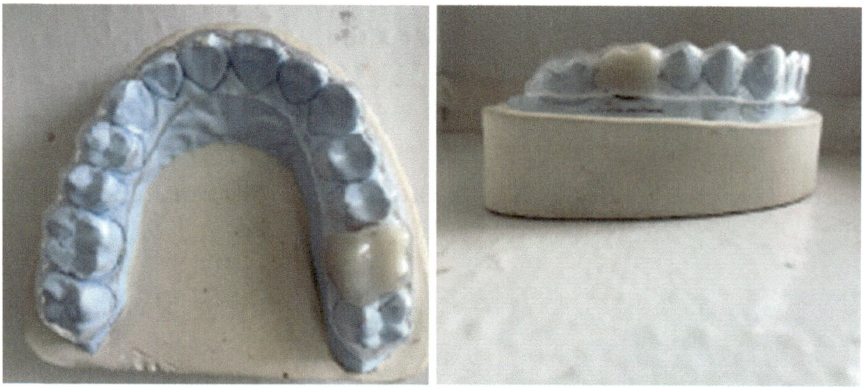

Fig. 13 Left picture: Occlusal view of the guide fixed on the cast, and the prosthetic position using composite flow. Right picture: Buccal view of the guide fixed on the cast and the prosthetic position using composite flow

higher accuracy, more time efficiency, easy to use, and higher acceptance rates from patients. The guides are made in two parts: the base and the tubes. Each implant system has its own guided surgical kits and drilling system. A practitioner should always follow the manufacturer's recommendation when using static guided surgical implant placements. The stability of the guide can be checked by placement on printed models or intraorally. Figure 15 presents a fully guided tooth-supported surgical stent made by stereolithography technique to place four implants.

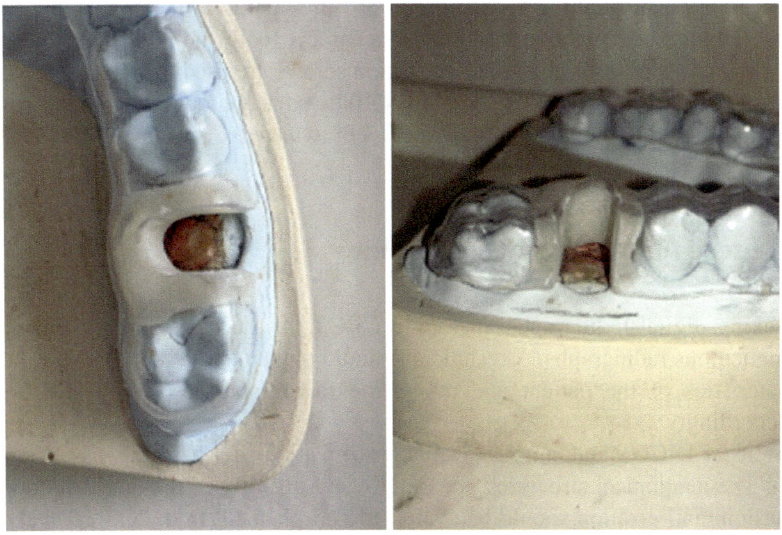

Fig. 14 Left picture: Occlusal view of access hole created for drilling purpose. Right picture: Buccal view of access hole created for drilling purpose

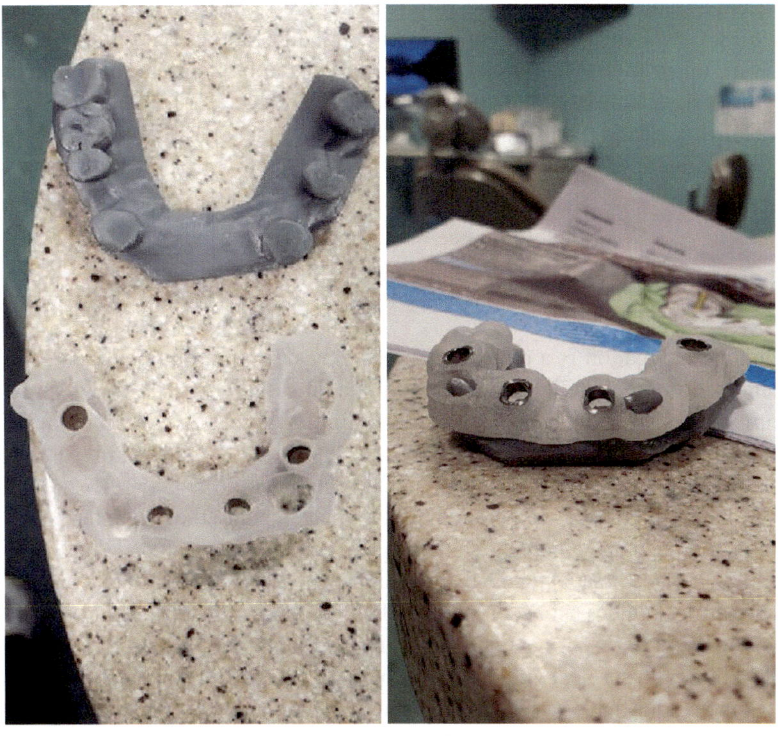

Fig. 15 Left picture: a printed model of a patient's mandibular teeth along with the surgical stent. Right picture: seated surgical guide on the printed model

The clinician should consider the following factors when proceeding with computer-guided implant series: CBCT accuracy, tooth mobility, number of the missing teeth, and restorative plans. Fixation screws are used to stabilize the guide intraorally for both tissue and bone guides. If the adjacent tooth or teeth are mobile, the guide should be extended to the other teeth to have the most stability.

10 Steps for Static Surgical Guide

1. Taking digital radiographs, including CBCT. An accurate surgery starts with meticulous radiographs. A technician should pay attention to the physical characteristics of the patient and adjust the radiographs, especially the CBCT, accordingly.
2. Transfer DICOM data into an available software for further analysis.

   The anatomical structures, the quality and quantity of the bone, the implant design, and position should be evaluated and planned. In the CBCT analyzing process, any pathologic or abnormality should be explained to the patient and addressed properly.
3. Record intraoral structures using an intraoral scanner or conventional impressions. Unaltered impressions are essential to have highly accurate surgical guides. The STL file is needed to proceed with implant planning. Merging two files, CBCT and STL files, aids to plan implant positions accordingly. Diagnostic wax up or digital restorative designs direct the clinician in making temporary restorative templates and an exact surgical guidance [22].
4. Delivery of the plan to the printer or milling machine. The practitioner should check the fit of the stent on the model before trying intraorally.

11 Dynamic Navigation

Dynamic navigation is a recent technology that is a micron tracker camera. It has been used in medical fields such as orthopedic surgery, maxillofacial surgery, and neurosurgery. It helps a surgeon to place implants with a high accuracy [23–25]. Dynamic navigation is considered an easy technique to learn and results in better time management for implant placement procedures [26].

Block et al. compared free-hand implant placement to the computer-guided navigation approach and computer static surgery guides. He concluded that the accuracy of implant placement using navigation surgery is superior to free-hand and similar to static surgical guides using computerized tomography scan [27]. Although researches show the superiority of navigation system over free-hand, the combination of using navigation with surgical guides receive higher accuracy over navigation alone [9].

Some studies have concluded that the dynamic navigation demonstrates 0.4 mm of entry error and 4 degree of implant angular deviation, but the success rate is similar to conventional drilling methods [28–30].

Table 2 Some benefits and indications of static surgical guide and dynamic navigation

Surgical guide	Benefits	Indication
Static surgical guide	1. Higher accuracy for implant position 2. Consuming less surgical time 3. Limiting clinician deviation 4. Avoiding trauma to adjacent anatomical structure	1. Flapless surgery 2. Aiding to make a bone reduction guide if needed 3. Assisting in fabricating a provisional crown out of CBCT generated guide 4. Full arch fixed crown and bridge, removable overdenture, STI, and hybrid dentures
Dynamic navigation	1. Consuming less clinical time 2. No need of impression 3. Involves less laboratory work 4. Avoiding trauma to adjacent anatomical structure 5. No need of laboratory work 6. More freedom for clinician to make adjustments at time of surgery 7. Cost-efficient	1. Patients with limited mouth opening 2. CBCT and implant placement at same appointment placement 3. Provide indirect vision 4. Not enough interocclusal space for static guides with tubes 5. Limited space close to natural tooth 6. Flap surgery, STI, multiple implants

It is imperative that the clinician avoids any tooth with mobility or temporary crowns for placement of clip arrays while registering the device [30].

Choosing the static CBCT-generated guides or dynamic navigation is based on clinician experience, preference, location of implant, surgical accessibility, and restorative plan. As practitioner's experience and surgical skills increase, the tendency for dynamic navigation increases due to cost-efficiency and more freedom of adjustment at time of surgery. Table 2 presents indications and benefits for the static surgical guide and dynamic navigation [30].

To date, the followings navigation systems are available for practitioners to utilize:

1. Navident navigation system (ClaroNav, claronav.com, Canada).
2. X-Guide navigation system (X-Nav, x-navtech.com, USA).
3. Image Dental implant (Image Navigation, image-navigation.com, Israel).
4. YOMI Navigation (Neocis, neocis.Com, USA).
5. Inliant Navigation (Navigate Surgical, navigatesurgical.com, Canada) [23].

12 Steps for Dynamic Navigation

1. Taking a CBCT.
2. Uploading DICOM data to the software.
3. Tracing important anatomical structures such as inferior alveolar nerve, mental nerve, maxillary sinus, and other structures.
4. Obtaining intraoral scans.
5. Uploading the scans to the software.

6. Superimpose intraoral scan with CBCT.
7. Plan virtual implant placement: selecting the right size, angulation, and depth.
8. Plan the final restoration for the future implant.
9. Coordinating the drill tip to the planned CBCT through tracking, registration, and calibration.
10. Implant placement according to the protocols.

Figures 16 and 17 are provided by Dr. Shaltoni, demonstrating implant placement by YOMI navigation.

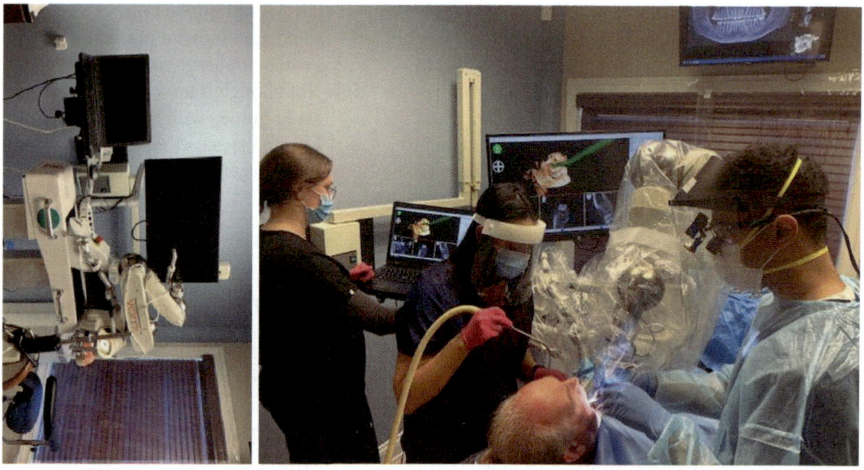

Fig. 16 YOMI navigation used by Samer Shaltoni DMD, MS to perform single implant placement #19 using the YOMI navigation system

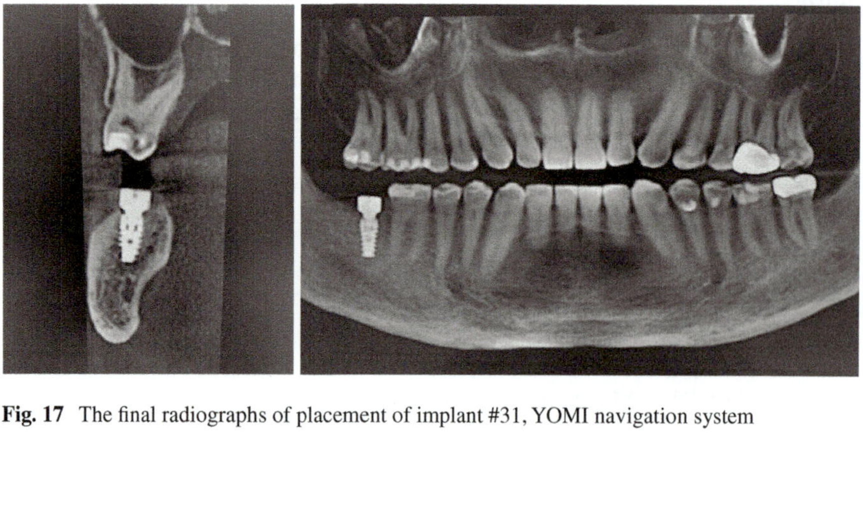

Fig. 17 The final radiographs of placement of implant #31, YOMI navigation system

13 Summary

Surgical guides are divided into fully guided or partially guided surgical stents. They can be fabricated by different methods. Today's technology aids clinicians to increase accuracy of implant placement while decreasing time and cost. Dynamic navigation is another useful system which provides practitioners more effective time and cost management as well as laboratory work. As mentioned in the chapter, dynamic navigation has its own indications and benefits. With thorough treatment planning, recent available advanced technology and choice of surgical stent, the implant outcome is more predictable.

References

1. Restorative driven implant solutions using the latest technology. Glidewell. https://glidewelldental.com/education/inclusive-dental-implant-magazine/volume-3-issue-1/restorative-driven-implant-solutions-utilizing-the-latest-technology/. Accessed 22 August 2021.
2. Poor implant placement causes its failure. Elite prosthetic dentistry. https://www.eliteprostheticdentistry.com/poor-implant-placement-causes-its-failure/. Published 13 May 2013. Accessed 15 August 2021.
3. Levin L. Dealing with dental implant failures. J Appl Oral Sci. 2008;16(3):171–5. https://doi.org/10.1590/S1678-77572008000300002.
4. Stevens MR, Ghasemi S, Tabrizi R, editors. Innovative perspectives in oral and maxillofacial surgery. Cham: Springer International Publishing; 2021. https://doi.org/10.1007/978-3-030-75750-2.
5. Manikandan RG. Implant surgical guides: from the past to the present. J Pharm Bioallied Sci. 2013;5(Suppl 1):S98. https://doi.org/10.4103/0975-7406.113306.
6. Cushen SE, Turkyilmaz I. Impact of operator experience on the accuracy of implant placement with stereolithographic surgical templates: an in vitro study. J Prosthet Dent. 2013;109(4):248–54. https://doi.org/10.1016/S0022-3913(13)60053-0.
7. Rosenfeld AL, Mandelaris GA, Tardieu PB. Prosthetically directed implant placement using computer software to ensure precise placement and predictable prosthetic outcomes. Part 1: diagnostics, imaging, and collaborative accountability. Restor Dent. 2005;26(3):8.
8. Orentlicher G, Horowitz A, Goldwaser B, Abboud M. Ten myths of guided implant surgery. Compend Contin Educ Dent. 2017;38(8):552–7.
9. Tm S, He L, Th L. Comparing accuracy of implant installation with a navigation system (NS), a laboratory guide (LG), NS with LG, and freehand drilling. Int J Environ Res Public Health. 2020;17(6):2107. https://doi.org/10.3390/ijerph17062107.
10. Shelley AM, Ferrero A, Brunton P, Goodwin M, Horner K. The impact of CBCT imaging when placing dental implants in the anterior edentulous mandible: a before–after study. Dentomaxillofac Radiol. 2015;44(4):20140316. https://doi.org/10.1259/dmfr.20140316.
11. Al Yafi F, Camenisch B, Al-Sabbagh M. Is digital guided implant surgery accurate and reliable? Dent Clin N Am. 2019;63(3):381–97. https://doi.org/10.1016/j.cden.2019.02.006.
12. Wood R, Sun Z, Chaudhry J, Tee BC, Kim D-G, Leblebicioglu B, England G. Factors affecting the accuracy of buccal alveolar bone height measurements from cone-beam computed tomography images. Am J Orthod Dentofacial Orthop. 2013;143(3):353–63. https://doi.org/10.1016/j.ajodo.2012.10.019.

13. Koch GK, Hamilton A, Wang K, et al. Dimensional accuracy of cone beam CT with varying angulation of the jaw to the X-ray beam. Dentomaxillofac Radiol. 2019;48(4):20180319. https://doi.org/10.1259/dmfr.20180319.
14. Kamburoğlu K. Use of dentomaxillofacial cone beam computed tomography in dentistry. World J Radiol. 2015;7(6):128. https://doi.org/10.4329/wjr.v7.i6.128.
15. Grimwood A, Thomas K, Kember S, Aldis G, Lawes R, Brigden B, Francis J, Henegan E, Kerner M, Delacroix L, Gordon A, Tree A, Harris EJ, McNair HA. Factors affecting accuracy and precision in ultrasound guided radiotherapy. Phys Imaging Radiat Oncol. 2021;18:68–77. https://doi.org/10.1016/j.phro.2021.05.003.
16. The glossary of prosthodontic terms. J Prosthet Dent. 2005;94:1. https://doi.org/10.1016/j.prosdent.2005.03.013.
17. Koyanagi K. Development and clinical application of a surgical guide for optimal implant placement. J Prosthet Dent. 2002;88(5):548–52. https://doi.org/10.1067/mpr.2002.129377.
18. Sahwil H. Choosing the right type of surgical guide or safe guide. https://blog.ddslab.com/type-of-surgical-guide-or-safe-guide. Accessed 27 August 2021.
19. Bencharit S, Staffen A, Yeung M, Whitley D 3rd, Laskin DM, Deeb GR. In vivo tooth-supported implant surgical guides fabricated with desktop stereolithographic printers: fully guided surgery is more accurate than partially guided surgery. J Oral Maxillofac Surg. 2018;76(7):1431–9. https://doi.org/10.1016/j.joms.2018.02.010.
20. CBCT: the new standard of care, are you getting the full picture? Integrated dental care. https://www.idcexton.com/blog/2020/october/cbct-the-new-standard-of-care-are-you-getting-th/. Accessed 22 August 2021.
21. Pattanaik S, Pattanaik BK. Fabrication of a surgical guide with help of a milling machine by ridge mapping method. J Indian Prosthodont Soc. 2013;13(1):61. https://doi.org/10.1007/s13191-012-0199-5.
22. Dandekeri SS, Sowmya MK, Bhandary S. Stereolithographic surgical template: a review. J Clin Diagn Res. 2013;7(9):2093. https://doi.org/10.7860/JCDR/2013/6052.3418.
23. Mandelaris GA, Stefanelli LV, DeGroot BS. Dynamic navigation for surgical implant placement: overview of technology, key concepts, and a case report. Compend Contin Educ Dent. 2018;39(9):614–21; quiz 622
24. Jayaratne YSN, Zwahlen RA, Lo J, Tam SC, Cheung LK. Computer-aided maxillofacial surgery: an update. Surg Innov. 2010;17(3):217–25. https://doi.org/10.1177/1553350610371626.
25. Luebbers HT, Messmer P, Obwegeser JA, et al. Comparison of different registration methods for surgical navigation in cranio-maxillofacial surgery. J Craniomaxillofac Surg. 2008;36(2):109–16. https://doi.org/10.1016/j.jcms.2007.09.002.
26. Pellegrino G, Bellini P, Cavallini PF, et al. Dynamic navigation in dental implantology: the influence of surgical experience on implant placement accuracy and operating time. An in vitro study. Int J Environ Res Public Health. 2020;17(6):2153. https://doi.org/10.3390/ijerph17062153.
27. EBSCOhost | 121352331 | Implant placement accuracy using dynamic navigation. Accessed 20 August 2021. https://web.b.ebscohost.com/abstract?direct=true&profile=ehost&scope=site&authtype=crawler&jrnl=08822786&asa=Y&AN=121352331&h=B239RhXEMpBaHjedtJo5NhoAfiQ9DKfY7d2s5pG88bIEPExGb50wLyG1ztIIptGpEUhFbZ1vgV%2fOTvwN6uq2%2fQ%3d%3d&crl=c&resultNs=AdminWebAuth&resultLocal=ErrCrlNotAuth&crlhashurl=login.aspx%3fdirect%3dtrue%26profile%3dehost%26scope%3dsite%26authtype%3dcrawler%26jrnl%3d08822786%26asa%3dY%26AN%3d121352331
28. Chiu W-K, Luk W-K, Cheung L-K. Three-dimensional accuracy of implant placement in a computer-assisted navigation system. Int J Oral Maxillofac Implants. 2006;21(3):465–70.
29. Kramer F-J, Baethge C, Swennen G, Rosahl S. Navigated vs. conventional implant insertion for maxillary single tooth replacement. Clin Oral Implants Res. 2005;16(1):60–8. https://doi.org/10.1111/j.1600-0501.2004.01058.x.
30. Block MS, Emery RW. Static or dynamic navigation for implant placement—choosing the method of guidance. J Oral Maxillofac Surg. 2016;74(2):269–77. https://doi.org/10.1016/j.joms.2015.09.022.

Index

S. A. Parhiz et al. (eds.), *Navigation in Oral and Maxillofacial Surgery*,
https://doi.org/10.1007/978-3-031-06223-0

GPSR Compliance

The European Union's (EU) General Product Safety Regulation (GPSR) is a set of rules that requires consumer products to be safe and our obligations to ensure this.

If you have any concerns about our products, you can contact us on ProductSafety@springernature.com

In case Publisher is established outside the EU, the EU authorized representative is:

Springer Nature Customer Service Center GmbH
Europaplatz 3
69115 Heidelberg, Germany

Batch number: 10732090

Printed by Printforce, the Netherlands